Delicious Diabetic Cookbook for Beginners:

2000+ Days Super Easy Recipes for Managing Prediabetes & Type 2 Diabetes. Includes 30-Day Meal Plan for Improved Healthy Habits Life

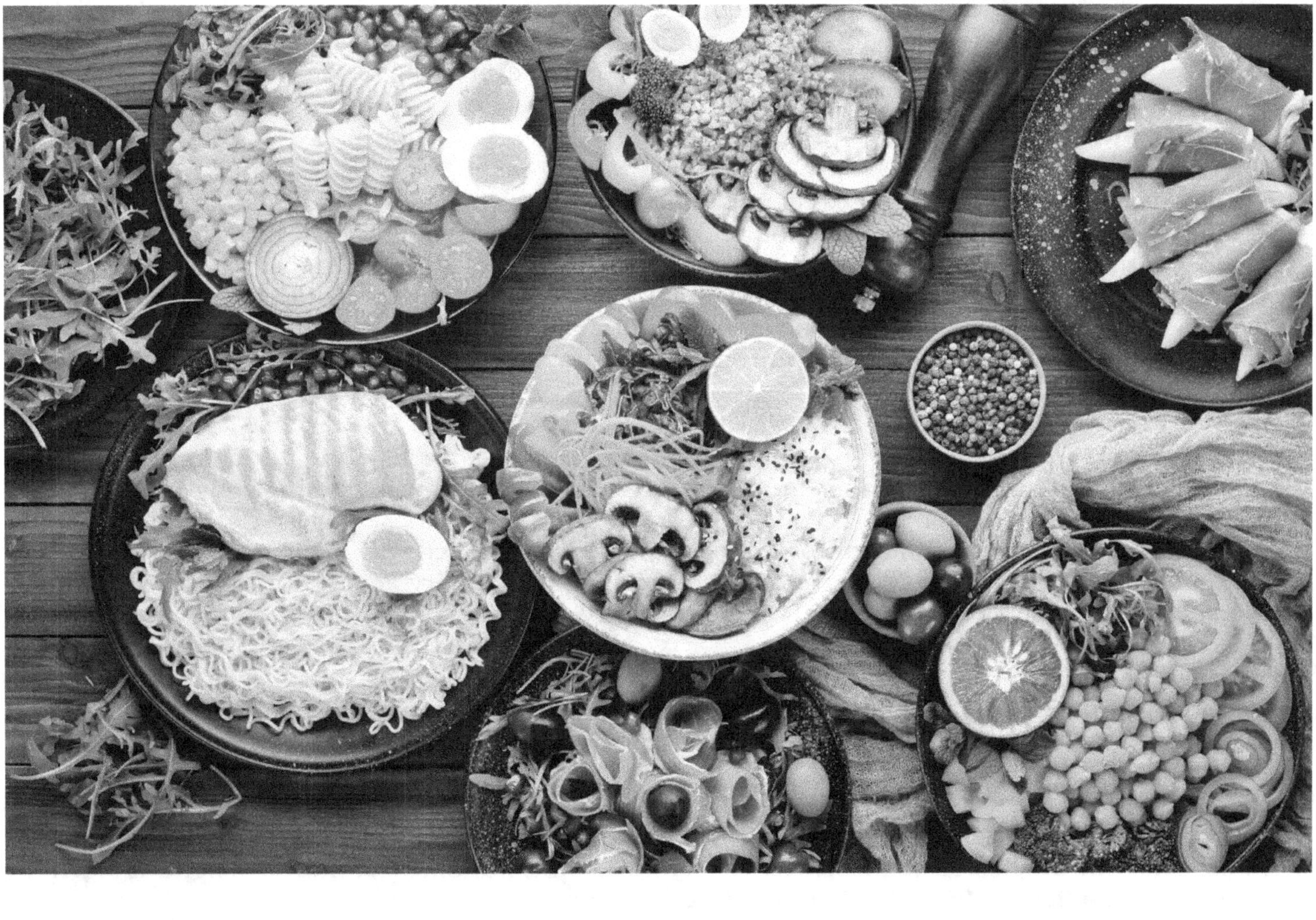

Amanda Kim

Embark on a unique and flavorful odyssey with the **"Delicious Diabetic Cookbook for Beginners: 2000+ Days Super Easy Recipes for Managing Prediabetes & Type 2 Diabetes."** This cookbook is not just a collection of Recipes but a beacon guiding you toward a healthier lifestyle. Crafted with love and a sprinkle of culinary magic, this tome of taste is presented "as is," a treasure chest of ideas and inspiration.

A Spoonful of Reality

The author and the publisher, akin to seasoned chefs blending ingredients, have meticulously compiled this collection with the utmost care and consideration. Yet, just as every palate is unique, so is the health and wellness journey. The information provided in this book is for educational purposes only and should not be considered medical advice or a substitute for professional healthcare consultation. Our recipes are stars in a vast dietary cosmos, meant to guide, not dictate, your path to wellness. We're here to support, guide, and help you make the best choices for your health. You're not alone in this journey; we're here with you every step of the way.

A Pinch of Caution

The delicious narratives and culinary compositions are intended solely for informational feasting. They are not designed to substitute for the professional advice offered by your healthcare sommelier. Our goal is to enlighten and inspire, not to provide medical diagnosis, treatment, cure, or prevention of any health issues. We advocate for a partnership with your healthcare provider to tailor these recipes to your health journey. Your health is our priority; we want you to feel safe and informed in your choices. Remember, your healthcare provider is your best ally in this journey.

A Dash of Personalized Wisdom

We understand the craving for change and the hunger for health, but seasoning your expectations with a touch of reality is essential. The success stories throughout these pages are the desserts, not the main course. They represent extraordinary outcomes, sweetened with hard work and dedication—flavors that may vary in the kitchen of life. Your culinary adventure will be your own, with results as diverse as the ingredients in your pantry.

By turning these pages, you're not just reading a book; you're seasoning your life with the possibility of transformation. The publisher and author are your companions on this voyage, offering insights and inspiration, but the ultimate creation—the improved you—is a dish only you can prepare.

Savor each recipe and each piece of advice with the understanding that this book is but one ingredient in your kitchen of wellness. Here's to your health, happiness, and the delightful journey that awaits in **"Delicious Diabetic Cookbook for Beginners."**

TABLE OF CONTENTS

INTRODUCTION

Welcome to a new chapter in your journey filled with hope, flavor, and the power to transform. Considering your challenges with prediabetes or type 2 diabetes, this book is crafted as a compassionate companion to guide you toward a brighter, healthier horizon. It's more than just a cookbook; it's a friend who understands the ups and downs, struggles, and triumphs of managing your health.

The Power of Food

Imagine a world where every meal is a step towards wellness, where delicious and nutritious dishes work harmoniously to stabilize your blood sugar levels and invigorate your overall health. Food is not just sustenance; it's a medicine, a source of joy, and a pathway to healing. Through the alchemy of wholesome ingredients and heartfelt cooking, we aim to show you how every bite can be a celebration of life and a testament to your resilience. Each recipe is a small victory, a step towards a healthier, happier you.

Setting the Stage

Gear up for a gastronomic journey that promises simplicity without sacrifice. This book unfolds a treasure trove of easy-to-follow recipes sprinkled with practical tips and garnished with wisdom to nourish body and soul. From the comfort of your home kitchen to the joy of a family dinner, we lay out a structured meal plan that fits seamlessly into your life, making healthy eating a pleasure, not a chore. Expect to find solace in the following pages, a guide that illuminates the path to managing your condition with grace and flavor. You'll find cooking for your health easy, enjoyable, and delicious.

Healthy Tips for Eating Out and Social Events

Venturing out into the world doesn't have to mean leaving your healthy habits at the door. We understand the importance of staying true to your journey, even in the face of tempting menus and social gatherings. With an arsenal of intelligent strategies for eating out and enjoying social events without compromise, this book gives you the confidence to make choices that align with your health goals. Because every celebration should feel inclusive, and every meal out should still feel like a step forward on your path to wellness.

Join us as we peel back the layers of doubt and uncertainty to reveal the vibrant potential within you. It's time to nourish not just your body but your spirit, too.

Together, let's savor the journey towards a life rich in health and happiness.

CHAPTER 1. UNDERSTANDING DIABETES MADE EASY

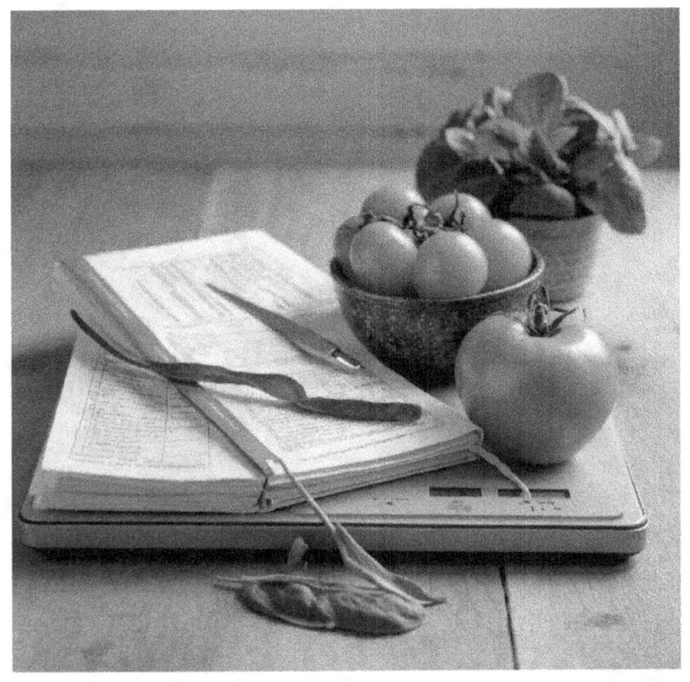

This section provides a glossary of crucial diabetes and nutrition terms to clarify and enrich your reading experience.

Welcome to your first journey towards understanding and managing diabetes efficiently and confidently. This chapter breaks down the basics, dusts off the complexities, and serves diabetes essentials on a silver platter.

WHAT IS DIABETES? LET'S MAKE IT SIMPLE

Explain prediabetes and type 2 diabetes, including symptoms and risk factors.

Imagine your body as a bustling city and glucose (sugar) as the energy that powers it. Now, insulin is the key that lets glucose into the city's cells to power up everything. In diabetes, it's like having rusty keys (Type 2) or losing them (Type 1), making it challenging for glucose to get where it needs to go. It leaves too much sugar floating around in your bloodstream, and just like in any city, too much of anything can cause problems.

Dive into the heart of understanding diabetes with a no-fuss, straightforward guide designed just for you. In **"Delicious Diabetic Cookbook for Beginners,"** we peel back the confusion surrounding diabetes and lay it out in bites you can easily digest. Here's a straightforward rundown on diabetes, broken down into easily understandable language:

Diabetes: The Basics

Imagine your body as a bustling metropolis and sugar (glucose) as the energy that powers its every corner. Insulin acts like the city's transportation system, helping sugar move from the bloodstream into the cells, where it's converted into energy. But sometimes, this system faces challenges:

- **Prediabetes:** The city's traffic lights are starting to malfunction. The sugar isn't moving as smoothly into the cells, leading to traffic jams in the bloodstream. This stage is a heads-up, signaling that without changes, full-blown diabetes could be around the corner.

- **Type 2 Diabetes**: The city's traffic system is significantly overwhelmed. The body either doesn't make enough insulin or can't use it efficiently, causing sugar to build up in the blood. This is the most common form of diabetes, and it's directly linked to lifestyle choices.

Symptoms to Watch Out For

Keep an eye out for the signs that the city's traffic flow might be off:

- **Feeling more thirsty than usual**
- **Frequent trips to the bathroom**
- **Feeling tired**
- **Blurred vision**
- **Cuts or wounds that heal slowly**

Risk Factors: Who's in the Driver's Seat?

Some folks are more likely to get caught in the traffic jam:

- **Being overweight**
- **A family history of diabetes**
- **Being 45 years or older**
- **Leading a sedentary lifestyle**
- **Having high blood pressure or cholesterol**

Understanding diabetes is critical to effective management. With **"Delicious Diabetic Cookbook for Beginners,"** you're not just getting a collection of recipes but embarking on a journey to a healthier you. You have the knowledge and tools you need to make intelligent decisions about your health.

Let's drive towards a healthier life, one delicious meal at a time.

So, let's conclude:

- Prediabetes is like the city's early warning system. It's when sugar levels are high but not high enough to be full-blown diabetes. Think of it as your body whispering, "Hey, something's up."
- Type 2 Diabetes means your body's insulin keys are malfunctioning. The doors to your cells don't open easily, resulting in elevated blood sugar levels.

KNOW YOUR NUMBERS: YOUR HEALTH DASHBOARD

Here, dear reader is a basic overview of blood sugar levels and the importance of monitoring for diabetes management.

Observing your blood sugar levels is like checking your car's dashboard. It tells you if your vehicle is running smoothly or if trouble is brewing.

Here's the scoop:

- **Blood Sugar Levels** are the main numbers to watch. They're like your health's speedometer, showing how much glucose is in your bloodstream.
- **Monitoring is critical** to managing diabetes. It's like regularly checking your car's oil level to avoid engine trouble down the road.

In **"Delicious Diabetic Cookbook for Beginners,"** we take the guesswork out of one of the most crucial aspects of managing diabetes: knowing and understanding your blood sugar levels. Let's break it down into bite-sized, easy-to-understand pieces that demystify the numbers game.

Blood Sugar Basics: Your Body's Energy Meter

Think of your body as a high-tech gadget. Just like a gadget needs a battery level indicator, your body has blood sugar levels to show how much energy you have available. These levels tell you if your energy is too low, just right, or too high.

Why Monitoring is Key

Observing your blood sugar is like checking the weather before heading out. It helps you make the best decisions for your day-to-day activities and meals. Here's why it's so crucial:

Dive into Chapter 2 of **"Delicious Diabetic Cookbook for Beginners"** and get ready to clear up all the carb confusion that's been clouding your mealtimes. We're about to lay down the basics of carbohydrates in the most straightforward, yummiest way possible, showing you how to make them your allies in managing diabetes. Let's break it down:

Carbohydrates: Your Body's Fuel

Imagine carbs as your body's favorite kind of fuel. Just as a car requires fuel, your body needs carbohydrates to energize. But not all fuel is created equal; the same goes for carbs.

The Good Guys: Complex Carbs

These carbs are the heroes of whole foods. You can find them in whole grains, fruits, vegetables, and beans. Think of them as slow-burning logs on a fire. They take their time to burn, supplying you with a continuous energy flow. This means your blood sugar levels rise gently, keeping you feeling full and energized longer.

The Not-So-Good Guys: Simple Carbs

Then there are the simple carbs that give carbs a bad name. These are the sugars and refined grains in sweets, white bread, and sodas. Like a pile of paper on fire, they burn up fast, causing your blood sugar to fluctuate wildly, soaring and plummeting like a roller coaster. This is not ideal for managing diabetes.

Why Carbs Matter for Blood Sugar

Grasping the distinction between healthy and unhealthy carbs is critical because it directly affects blood sugar control. It's not just about the quantity of carbs but the quality that matters.

- **Good carbs** = Smooth sailing: They help keep blood sugar levels stable, reducing the risk of spikes and making diabetes management easy.
- **Bad carbs** = Choppy waters: They can make your blood sugar levels spike and plummet, making it harder to control diabetes.

In **"Delicious Diabetic Cookbook for Beginners,"** we don't just preach; we guide you step by step with 2000+ days of super easy recipes. Each recipe is designed to embrace the good carbs while showing the door to the bad ones, all in a delicious way that doesn't make you feel like you're missing out.

So, get ready to say goodbye to carb confusion and hello to simple, delicious meals that help manage prediabetes and type 2 diabetes. Let's make every bite count towards a healthier, happier you!

- **Avoid Traffic Jams:** High blood sugar levels over time can lead to health problems, much like traffic jams can cause delays and frustration in our daily lives.
- **Keep the Energy Flowing:** Is your energy level too low? You might feel like you're running on empty. Keeping levels balanced ensures you have the right amount of energy.
- **Make Informed Choices:** Knowing your numbers helps tailor your meals and activities to maintain reasonable blood sugar control.

The Numbers Game: What's Normal, What's Not

Here's a simple guide: We measure blood sugar levels in milligrams per deciliter (mg/dL):

- **Fasting** (no eating for at least 8 hours): The average level is below 10here' dL. Prediabetes falls between 100 and 125 mg/dL, while diabetes starts at 126 mg/dL or above.
- **2 Hours After Eating:** Most people should be under 140 mg/dL.

Tools of the Trade

To keep track, you might use:

- **A Blood Glucose Meter:** A small, portable gadget that measures how much sugar is in your blood at any moment.
- **Continuous Glucose Monitoring** (CGM): A wearable device that provides real-time readings, offering a bigger picture of your blood sugar trends.

Monitoring your blood sugar is like having a personal road map for managing diabetes. It guides your food choices and activities and helps you navigate towards a healthier life. With our Cookbook, you will learn how to keep your numbers in check and enjoy the journey with delicious, diabetes-friendly recipes.

Let's take control of your health, one tasty meal and number at a time.

Lifestyle Matters: Steering Towards Health

This section offers practical diet, exercise, stress management, and sleep tips, which can affect blood sugar control and overall well-being. It also highlights the benefits of regular exercise in managing diabetes, including improved insulin sensitivity and weight management.

Your lifestyle is the driver's seat when it comes to controlling diabetes.

Here's how to take the wheel:

- **Diet:** Imagine your body as a high-performance vehicle. You want to fuel it with the best stuff. Foods low in sugar and high in nutrients are your premium fuel.

- **Exercise:** This is like giving your car a regular spin. It helps burn off excess fuel (sugar) and keeps the engine (your heart) running smoothly.

- **Stress Management:** Too much stress is like putting the wrong fuel in your car. Learning to chill can help keep your sugar levels in check.

- **Sleep:** Think of sleep as your car's nightly maintenance check. Quality shut-eye helps regulate sugar levels and repairs your body.

In **"Delicious Diabetic Cookbook for Beginners,"** we dive into the sweet life—not just through mouth-watering recipes but by mastering the art of living well. Chapter 1 isn't just about what's on your plate; it's about painting a bigger picture of health beyond the kitchen. Let's unwrap the lifestyle elements that can turn the tide in managing diabetes, making each day a masterpiece of well-being.

Fueling Up Right: The Power of Diet

Think of your body as a car. Just like premium fuel can make a car run smoothly, the right foods can keep your blood sugar levels in a sweet spot. Here's the deal:

- **Whole, Unprocessed Foods:** Eat plenty of veggies, lean proteins, and whole grains. They're like high-quality fuel that burns clean and steady.

- **Smart Swaps:** Choose complex carbs over simple sugars. It's like opting for a long-lasting battery instead of a quick-drain one.

Moving More: Exercise as Your Secret Weapon

Exercise isn't just about losing weight; it's like a direct conversation with your cells, telling them to open up and let sugar in, lowering your blood sugar naturally. Whether it's a brisk walk, a dance session, or yoga, moving more is about:

- **Boosting Insulin Sensitivity**: Making your body's insulin work better.

- **Energy and Mood Lift: Like** hitting the refresh button on your mood and energy levels.

The Chill Factor: Stress Management

Stress is like having a foot on your car's accelerator; it speeds up your blood sugar. Finding ways to relax is crucial:

- **Deep breathing or meditation:** These are your brakes that slow down the stress response.

- **Hobbies or Activities:** Engaging in things you love is like switching lanes from the fast-paced stress highway to a scenic, peaceful road.

Restful Nights: Sleep's Role in Blood Sugar Balance

Imagine your body does its maintenance work at night. Not getting enough sleep is like skipping essential repairs. Here's why zzz's matter:

- **Regulating Hormones:** A good night's sleep helps keep the hormones that affect your appetite and blood sugar in check.

- **Energy Recharge:** Quality sleep is like plugging in your body's battery for a full charge.

In **"Delicious Diabetic Cookbook for Beginners,"** we stitch these lifestyle threads into a tapestry of tips and tricks that can guide you to a healthier, happier life with diabetes. It's about making small changes that add up, turning healthy choices into habits, and habits into a lifestyle that powers your best life. Let's embark on this journey together, one step, one bite, one breath at a time.

Let's rev up your health engine and cruise towards a healthier life!

THE BONUS OF CHAPTER 1: GLOSSARY OF CRUCIAL DIABETES AND NUTRITION TERMS

Here's a meticulously crafted glossary for the **"Delicious Diabetic Cookbook for Beginners."** This comprehensive resource ensures you clearly understand all critical terms about diabetes and nutrition.

- **A1C (HbA1c)**: A rapid blood test that reveals your average blood sugar concentrations for the past three months. It helps you understand how well your diabetes is being managed.
- **Carbohydrates:** Often found in foods like bread, fruits, and sweets, these nutrients break down into glucose, which your body uses for energy. Managing how much you eat is critical for controlling blood sugar.
- **Diabetes:** A health condition where the body has trouble managing blood sugar levels. Type 1 diabetes is when the body can't make enough insulin, and Type 2 diabetes is when the body doesn't use insulin well.
- **Fiber:** A part of plant foods that the body can't digest. Plenty of fiber helps control blood sugar levels and keeps your digestive system healthy.
- **Glycemic Index (GI):** A tool that rates how different foods affect blood sugar levels. Foods with a high GI increase blood sugar more than foods with a low GI.
- **Insulin:** A vital hormone that converts glucose into energy and stabilizes blood sugar levels. The pancreas produces insulin, which is necessary for the body to use glucose for energy. In people with diabetes, the body either doesn't make enough insulin or doesn't use it effectively.
- **Macronutrients:** The ample three nutrients, carbohydrates, proteins, and fats, give your body energy.
- **Micronutrients:** Vital vitamins and minerals are needed in small quantities for optimal health and proper body function.
- **Prediabetes**: A warning sign where blood sugar levels are high but not high enough to be called diabetes. It's a wake-up call to start taking your health seriously.
- **Protein:** A crucial nutrient for building muscles and repairing tissues. Unlike carbs, protein has little effect on blood sugar.
- **Saturated Fats:** Fats from animal products can raise cholesterol, making heart disease more likely.
- **Unsaturated Fats:** Healthier fats found in plants and fish that help lower your cholesterol and protect your heart.
- **Whole Grains:** Grains that include the entire grain kernel. They have more nutrients and fiber than grains that have been refined.
- **30-Day Meal Plan: A** daily guide to monthly meals to kickstart healthier eating habits. It's beneficial for managing diabetes with diet.

This glossary uses straightforward language to explain terms related to diabetes and nutrition. It is a practical guide that instills confidence in your ability to make informed dietary choices as you navigate our cookbook.

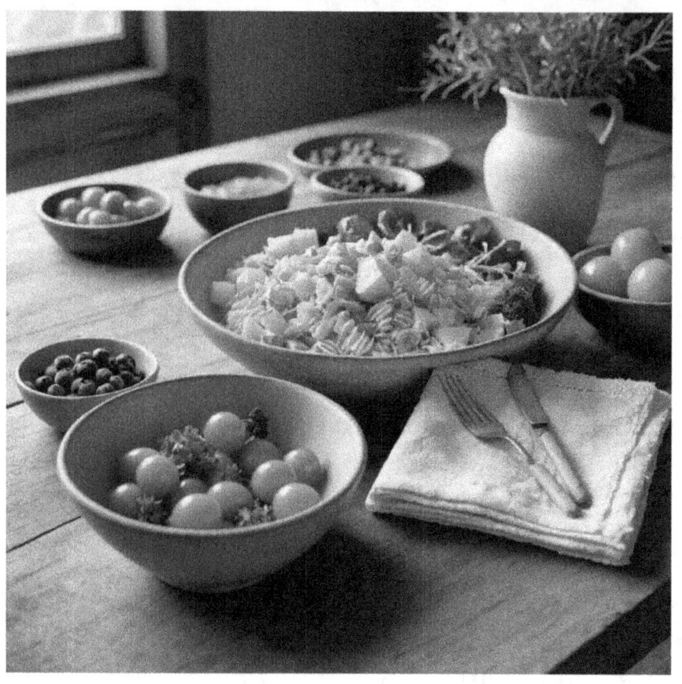

Chapter 2: The ABCs of Diabetes Nutrition:

Carb Confusion Cleared: Your Guide Through the Maze

Explain carbohydrates, including good vs. bad carbs, and how they impact blood sugar.

This section clearly explains carbohydrates, including the difference between 'good carbs' (complex carbohydrates that are slowly digested and do not induce a swift elevation in glucose levels) and 'bad carbs' (simple carbohydrates that are swiftly metabolized and may trigger a quick increase in glucose levels).

This Chapter serves up a tasty slice of knowledge on the ABCs of Diabetes Nutrition, focusing on demystifying carbs - often the most misunderstood characters on your plate. Let's break it down into bite-sized, easy-to-digest info that'll change how you look at your meals.

Carb Confusion Cleared:

Carbohydrates, or carbs, are fuel for our bodies' engines. But not all carbs are created equal. Think of them as guests at a party: some you're thrilled to see, and others you might wish had RSVP'd no.

Here's how to tell them apart:

- **Good Carbs (The Life of the Party):** These are whole, unprocessed foods like fruits, vegetables, whole grains, and legumes. They pack a lot of fiber, taking longer to break down. This slow burn keeps your blood sugar levels stable, like a steady, smooth playlist that keeps the party going without sudden crashes.

- **Bad Carbs (Party Crashers):** These are the refined or processed carbohydrates in white bread, pastries, and sugary beverages. They're stripped of their nutritional value and fiber, leading to a sharp rise and sudden drop in blood sugar levels—akin to a party crasher who spikes the punch and leaves you with the aftermath.

Why Carbs Matter in Diabetes Management

Understanding carbs is critical since they directly influence your blood sugar levels. Here's the lowdown:

- **Blood Sugar Balance:** By choosing good carbs over bad, you can help maintain a more consistent blood sugar level, avoiding those highs and lows that can make diabetes more complicated to manage.

- **Energy and Wellness:** Good carbs are nutrient-dense and vital for overall health and well-being.

"Delicious Diabetic Cookbook for Beginners" doesn't just stop at explaining carbs; it shows you how to incorporate them wisely into your diet, with recipes crafted to tantalize your taste buds while managing your blood sugar levels. It's about enjoying a wide range of foods without the guilt, armed with the knowledge to make choices that support your health journey. Let's turn the page on carb confusion and embrace the delicious, nutritious world of diabetes-friendly eating.

Get ready to clear up all the carb confusion clouding your mealtimes. We're about to lay down the basics of carbohydrates in the most straightforward, yummiest way possible, showing you how to make them your allies in managing diabetes. Let's break it down:

Carbohydrates: Your Body's Fuel

Imagine carbs as your body's favorite kind of fuel. Just as a car requires fuel, your body needs carbohydrates for energy. But not all fuel is created equal; the same goes for carbs.

The Good Guys: Complex Carbs

These carbs are the heroes of whole foods. They are found in whole grains, fruits, vegetables, and beans. Think of them as the slow-burning logs on a fire; they take their time to burn, offering you a consistent energy supply. This means your blood sugar levels rise gently, keeping you feeling full and energized longer.

The Not-So-Good Guys: Simple Carbs

Then there are the simple carbs that give carbs a bad name. These are the sugars and refined grains in sweets, white bread, and sodas. Like a pile of paper on fire, they burn up fast, causing your blood sugar to oscillate dramatically, with sharp increases and sudden declines. This is not ideal for managing diabetes.

Why Carbs Matter for Blood Sugar

It is critical to learn to distinguish between beneficial and harmful carbohydrates because they directly impact your blood sugar control. It's not just about the quantity of carbs but the quality that matters.

- **Good carbs = Smooth sailing:** They help keep blood sugar levels stable, reducing the risk of spikes and making diabetes management easy.
- **Bad carbs = Choppy waters:** They can make your blood sugar levels spike and plummet, making it harder to control diabetes.

In **"Delicious Diabetic Cookbook for Beginners,"** we don't just preach; we accompany you at every step with 2000+ days of super easy recipes. Each recipe is designed to embrace the good carbs while showing the door to the bad ones, all in a delicious way that doesn't make you feel like you're missing out.

So, get ready to say goodbye to carb confusion and hello to simple, delicious meals that help manage prediabetes and type 2 diabetes. **Let's make every bite count towards a healthier, happier you.**

Step into Chapter 2 of **"Delicious Diabetic Cookbook for Beginners,"** where we unravel the magic behind Portion Power. Mastering portion control is like finding the perfect balance on a seesaw, ensuring everything is correct.

Let's break down this essential skill into fun, manageable steps that'll transform how you eat, one plate at a time.

Simple portion control guidelines to help manage blood sugar levels and sustain a healthy weight.

Imagine your plate is a canvas, and portion control is your brush. With it, you can paint the perfect nutritional picture that helps manage your blood sugar levels and keeps your weight in check.

Here's how to make portion control your secret ingredient to a healthier life:

Use Your Hands as a Guide

- Proteins (think meats, tofu): Size of your palm
- Carbohydrates (like rice, pasta): Fist-sized
- Vegetables: As much as you can hold in both hands
- Fats (nuts, oils): Thumb-sized

This method is as simple as it gets, turning your hands into the most portable measuring tools ever!

The Plate Method: A Visual Guide

Picture your plate divided into three parts:

- Half of it is filled with colorful veggies (the more, the merrier!)
- One quarter with lean protein (keeping it varied from fish to beans)
- The final quarter should include whole grains or starchy vegetables (think quinoa, sweet potatoes)

Listen to Your Body

Eating slowly and mindfully lets your body catch up to your brain, signaling when you're full. It's like checking in with a friend during a meal, ensuring you enjoy the experience without overdoing it.

Meal Prep: Portion Control's Best Friend

Meal Prep: Portion Control's Best Friend Preparing your meals in advance is not just a time-saver; it's a portion controller's paradise. It allows you to precisely determine how much to eat, keeping those portions in check before hunger takes over.

In **"Delicious Diabetic Cookbook for Beginners,"** we take the guesswork out of portion control with 2000+ days of super easy recipes designed with balance. From hearty breakfasts to satisfying dinners, our 30-Day Meal Plan demonstrates how to integrate portion control effortlessly into a diabetes-friendly lifestyle.

Say goodbye to weighing and measuring. Say hello to simple visual cues that make eating right a breeze. Let's embrace Portion Power together, making every meal an opportunity to fuel your body ideally.

THE BONUS OF CHAPTER 2: BALANCED PLATE

Quick tips to make meals with the right mix of protein, healthy fats, fiber, and carbs.

Creating a balanced plate is like being an artist with your nutrition, painting a masterpiece of health with every meal. In **"Delicious Diabetic Cookbook for Beginners,"** we dive into balancing your plate with protein, healthy fats, fiber, and carbohydrates. Let's explore how to craft these nutritional works of art with simple, easy-to-follow guidelines.

The Foundation: Divide Your Plate. Picture your plate as a canvas divided into three harmonious sections:

- **Half the Plate:** Vegetables. **Fill this space** with a rainbow of veggies to get nutrients and plenty of fiber. Think leafy greens, bright bell peppers, and everything in between.

- **One-Quarter of the Plate:** Protein

  This section is for your **proteins,** which are like the building blocks of your body. Choose lean options like skinless chicken breast, fish, tofu, or beans. These power players keep you feeling full and satisfied.

- **The Remaining Quarter:** Carbohydrates

  Carbs are your body's primary energy source. Choose whole grains like brown rice, quinoa, whole-wheat pasta, or starchy vegetables like sweet potatoes. They deliver long-lasting energy and are rich in fiber.

Adding Color and Texture: Fruits and Healthy Fats

- **Fruits:** While not always on the plate, fruits are great for adding a sweet touch to meals or serving as a healthy snack. They are packed with plenty of vitamins, minerals, and fiber.

- **Healthy Fats:** Drizzle olive oil over your veggies, add avocado slices to your meal, or sprinkle nuts or seeds for crunch. Healthy fats help absorb vitamins and keep you feeling full.

The Secret Ingredient: Water

- **Stay Hydrated:** Accompany your balanced plate with a glass of water. Staying hydrated is crucial for digestion, nutrient absorption, and overall health. It also helps regulate blood levels of sugar and supports weight management.

Meal Building Blocks:

- **Start with Vegetables:** Begin planning your meal by choosing vegetables to fill half your plate.
- **Pick Your Protein:** Decide on a lean protein to take up one-quarter of your plate.
- **Choose Your Carbs:** Select a whole-grain or starchy vegetable for the remaining quarter.
- **Add Healthy Fats:** Finish your meal with healthy fats for flavor and nutrition.
- **Remember Fruit:** Consider a side of fruit or incorporate it into your meal or dessert.

In the Delicious Diabetic Cookbook for Beginners, we guide you through 2000+ days of perfectly balanced meals, combining proteins, healthy fats, fiber, and carbohydrates to manage prediabetes and Type 2 diabetes effectively. With our 30-Day Meal Plan, you'll learn how to make balanced plates a natural part of your everyday life, leading to improved healthy habits for life.

Let's make every meal a balanced celebration of flavor and nutrition!

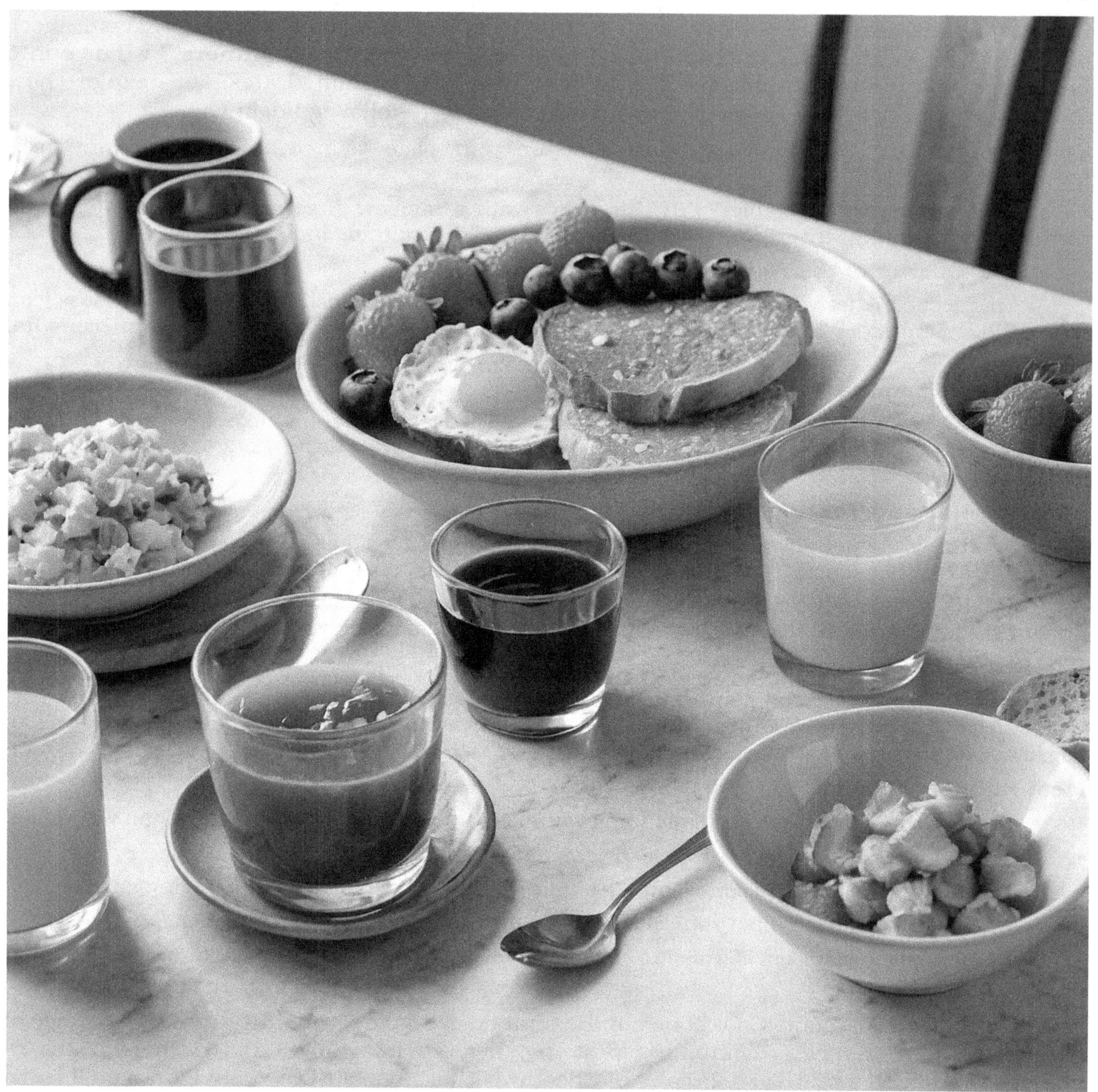

Rise and Shine with Breakfast

These mouth-watering breakfast recipes are quick to make and. maintain stable blood sugar levels throughout the morning.

Set off on a tasty adventure towards health with **Breakfast** in **"Delicious Diabetic Cookbook for Beginners."** Kickstart your mornings with zero added sugar, transforming breakfast into a celebration of taste and wellness.

Let's dive into a world where breakfast is not just the first meal of the day but the beginning of a healthier you.

MEDITERRANEAN SHAKSHUKA

Ingredients

- 1 tablespoon olive oil (a liquid embrace)
- 1 large onion, diced (the base of sweetness)
- 1 bell pepper, diced (a crunch of color)
- 2 cloves garlic, minced (a whisper of aroma)
- 1 teaspoon ground cumin (a dusting of the earth)
- 1 teaspoon smoked paprika (a smoky hug)
- 2 cups canned tomatoes, crushed (the essence of the garden)
- 4 large eggs (the stars of the show)
- 1/2 cup feta cheese, crumbled (the salty kiss)
- Salt and pepper, to taste (the balancing act)
  Fresh parsley or cilantro for garnish (a green flourish)

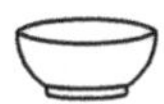  

Prep Time: 10 min   Cook Time: 20 min   Serves: 4

Directions

1. **Foundation of Flavor:** Heat the olive oil in a large skillet over medium heat. Add the onion and bell pepper, sauté until soft and sweet, for about 5 minutes. Stir in the garlic, cumin, and paprika, and let them dance together for a minute more.
2. **The Tomato Canvas:** Pour the crushed tomatoes and season with salt and pepper. Simmer the sauce until it thickens beautifully, about 10 minutes, painting a backdrop for your eggs.
3. **Nestle the Eggs:** Create little pockets in the sauce with a spoon and carefully crack an egg into each one. Place the lid on the skillet and allow the eggs to cook until they become firm, but the yolks remain delightfully creamy and runny, around 7-10 minutes.
4. **Final Touches:** Sprinkle with crumbled feta cheese and garnish with fresh parsley or cilantro. Serve hot, inviting each spoonful to be a journey to the Mediterranean.

Nutritional Information:

Per serving: Estimated values: 250 calories, 12g protein, 15g carbohydrates, 17g fat, 4g fiber, 210mg cholesterol, 320mg sodium, 450mg potassium.

Summary:

Savor the vibrant essence of the **Mediterranean** with this **Shakshuka**, a warm, spiced tomato sauce cradling poached eggs, finished with fresh herbs for a zesty twist. Perfect for any meal, it's a nourishing dance of flavors that brings a piece of the Mediterranean to your table.

=

Peanut Butter Banana Bowl

Ingredients

- 2 bananas, peeled and sliced (sweet and creamy)
- 2 tablespoons creamy peanut butter (rich and nutty)
- 1 cup almond milk (for a smooth blend)
- 1 tablespoon of dark chocolate shavings (for a decadent touch)

Nutritional Information:

Per serving: Estimated values: 310 calories, 8g protein, 44g carbohydrates, 14g fat, 6g fiber, 0mg cholesterol, 200mg sodium, 700mg potassium.

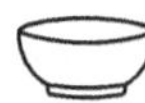  

Prep Time: 5 min   Cook Time: 0 min   Serves: 2

Directions

1. **Blend to Perfection:** In a blender, combine bananas, peanut butter, and almond milk. Blend until you achieve a smooth and creamy consistency.
2. **Serve It Up:** Pour the smoothie mixture into two bowls, dividing evenly.
3. **Garnish with Chocolate:** Sprinkle each bowl with dark chocolate shavings, adding a luxurious twist to your nutritious bowl.

Summary:

Dive into the **Peanut Butter Banana Bowl**, where every spoonful is a harmonious blend of creamy, nutty, and sweet flavors, crowned with the decadent indulgence of dark chocolate. This bowl is not just breakfast; it's a treat, promising to start your day on a deliciously high note.

Antioxidant Acai Bowl

Ingredients

- 2 packets (200 grams) of frozen acai berry puree (the superhero of antioxidants)
- one banana, sliced (for natural sweetness and creaminess)
- 1/2 cup mixed berries (blueberries, raspberries, and strawberries for a berry bonanza)
- 1/4 cup almond milk (to blend it all smoothly)
- 2 tablespoons sliced almonds (for a satisfying crunch)
- A dash of cinnamon (for a warm, spicy note)

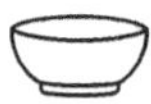  

Prep Time: 10 min   Cook Time: 0 min   Serves: 2

Directions

1. **Blend the Base:** Break the acai puree into your blender, add the banana and almond milk, and blend until smooth. If it's too thick, add a splash of almond milk.
2. **Pour It Out:** Evenly divide the acai mixture into two bowls, creating a velvety purple canvas.
3. **Top It Off:** Artfully arrange the mixed berries on top, sprinkle with sliced almonds, and finish with a dash of cinnamon for that extra zing.

Nutritional Information:

Per serving: Estimated values: 215 calories, 4g protein, 35g carbohydrates, 9g fat, 7g fiber, 0mg cholesterol, 15mg sodium, 250mg potassium.

Summary:

Welcome to the **Antioxidant Acai Bowl**, a vibrant start to your day packed with nutrients and flavors that dance on your palate. Each bite is a blend of creamy, crunchy, sweet, and spicy, ensuring your breakfast is as delightful as it is nutritious. Here's to a bowl full of wellness and zest!

HEARTY OATMEAL CREATIONS

Ingredients

- Cinnamon Apple Oatmeal: Rolled oats with stewed cinnamon apples and a sprinkle of walnuts.
- Berry Almond Overnight Oats: Overnight oats with mixed berries and a crunchy almond topping
- Pumpkin Spice Oatmeal: Warm oats with pumpkin puree, spice, and pecan pieces.
- Savory Oatmeal with Avocado: Oats cooked in vegetable broth, topped with sliced avocado and a poached egg.
- Chocolate Hazelnut Oatmeal: Cocoa-infused oats with hazelnuts and strawberries.

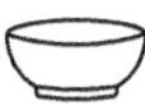  

Prep Time: 5 min   Cook Time: 0 min   Serves: 2

Directions

1. **Blend to Perfection:** Combine bananas, peanut butter, and almond milk in a blender. Blend until smooth.
2. **Serve It Up:** Pour the smoothie mixture into two bowls, dividing evenly.
3. **Garnish with Chocolate:** Sprinkle each bowl with dark chocolate shavings, adding a luxurious twist to your nutritious bowl.

Nutritional Information

Per serving: Estimated values: 300 calories, 10g protein, 45g carbohydrates, 12g fat, 8g fiber, 0mg cholesterol, 20mg sodium, 300mg potassium

Summary:

Easy way to provide a significant energy boost to power you through the day. Oats aren't just a breakfast staple here; they're the base for a parade of flavors, textures, and nourishments. Craft **Hearty Oatmeal Creations** recipes to kickstart your day with warmth and wellness.

CINNAMON APPLE OATMEAL

Ingredients

- 1 cup rolled oats (a hearty base)
- 2 cups water or milk (for creaminess)
- 1 large apple, peeled and diced (a crisp autumn harvest)
- 1 teaspoon of ground cinnamon (a warm spice embrace)
- 2 tablespoons walnuts, chopped (a crunchy finale)
- Optional sweeteners: honey, maple syrup, or brown sugar (to taste)

Nutritional Information:

Per serving: Estimated values: 180 calories, 3g protein, 23g carbohydrates, 9g fat, 4g fiber, 0mg cholesterol, 10mg sodium, 300mg potassium.

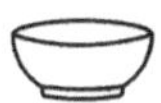  

Prep Time: 5 min   Cook Time: 0 min   Serves: 2

Directions

1. **Simmer Oats:** Cook oats according to package instructions.
2. **Cook Apples:** While oats cook, sauté apples in a pan with cinnamon until soft.
3. **Combine and Serve:** Mix cooked apples and walnuts into the prepared oatmeal. Drizzle with honey for added sweetness.
4. **Serve Warm:** This comforting bowl is perfect for starting the day or as a wholesome snack.

Summary:

Start your day with the comforting warmth of our **Cinnamon Apple Oatmeal**, a blend of hearty oats, sweet and tart apples, and a hint of cinnamon. This delightful treat satisfies your cravings for something sweet and offers a nutritious beginning to your day.

GREEN GODDESS BOWL

Ingredients

- 2 cups spinach (a green powerhouse)
- 1 avocado, peeled and pitted (for creamy goodness)
- 1 green apple, cored and chopped (a crisp, tart twist)
- 1/4 cup pumpkin seeds (for a crunchy finish)

Nutritional Information:

Per serving: Estimated values: 290 calories, 5g protein, 30g carbohydrates, 20g fat, 10g fiber, 0mg cholesterol, 30mg sodium, 800mg potassium.

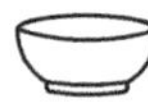  

Prep Time: 10 min   Cook Time: 0 min   Serves: 2

Directions

1. **Blend the Greens**: In your blender, combine the spinach, avocado, and green apple with a splash of water if needed. Blend until smooth and gloriously green.
2. **Pour and Prep:** Distribute the puree evenly into two bowls, creating a vibrant green base.
3. **Garnish Galore:** Sprinkle each bowl with pumpkin seeds, which will add texture and a nutty flavor to your nutrient-packed bowl.

Summary:

Welcome to a bowl so green and lush it's like diving into nature's treasure chest. The **Green Goddess Bowl** celebrates all things vibrant and nourishing, promising to leave you feeling rejuvenated and ready to take on the world.

CHOCOLATE HAZELNUT OATMEAL

Ingredients

- 1 cup rolled oats (the cozy canvas)
- 2 cups milk or water (for a silky or light texture)
- two tablespoons cocoa powder (a rich chocolate hug)
- 1/4 cup hazelnuts, roughly chopped (a nutty crunch)
- 1/2 cup strawberries, sliced (sweet, juicy kisses)
- Optional: sweetener of choice to taste (a whisper of sweetness)

Nutritional Information:

Per serving: Estimated values: 320 calories, 10g protein, 46g carbohydrates, 12g fat, 7g fiber, 0mg cholesterol, 50mg sodium, 400mg potassium

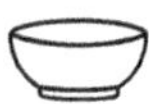  

Prep Time: 5 min   Cook Time: 10 min   Serves: 2

Directions

1. **Whisk in the Chocolate:** In a saucepan, bring the milk (or water) to a gentle simmer. Whisk in the cocoa powder until smooth. Stir in the oats and cook over medium heat, stirring occasionally, until the oats are tender and have absorbed the liquid, about 10 minutes.
2. **Toast the Hazelnuts:** While the oats cook, lightly toast the chopped hazelnuts in a dry skillet over medium heat until fragrant, for about 3 minutes, and observe to prevent burning.
3. **Make it Your Own**: Once the oatmeal is cooked, remove it from the heat and sweeten it to your liking. Whether you prefer the natural sweetness of honey, the rich depth of maple syrup, or the classic touch of sugar, the choice is yours to make this dish truly yours.
4. **Garnish and Enjoy:** Spoon the oatmeal into bowls and top with toasted hazelnuts and fresh strawberry slices.

Summary:

Let each spoonful of **Chocolate Hazelnut Oatmeal** transport you to a place of blissful indulgence, where the rich dance of cocoa and hazelnuts meets the sweet charm of strawberries. It's more than a meal; it's a moment of joy, a delightful escape to savor amidst the rush of the day.

VEGGIE OMELETTE

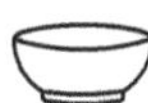

Prep Time: 5 min

Cook Time: 15 min

Serves: 2

Ingredients

- 4 large eggs (a canvas of protein)
- 1 cup fresh spinach (a handful of green vitality)
- 1/2 cup mushrooms, sliced (earthy treasures)
- 1/2 cup tomatoes, diced (juicy gems)
- Salt and pepper, to taste (the seasoning of life)
- 1 tablespoon of olive oil (for that silky smoothness)

Nutritional Information:

Per serving: Estimated values: 250 calories, 14g protein, 6g carbohydrates, 18g fat, 2g fiber, 370mg cholesterol, 220mg sodium, 400mg potassium.

Directions

1. **Get Mixing:** In a bowl, beat the eggs with a whisk, salt, and pepper until light and frothy, setting the stage for your veggie spectacle.
2. **Sauté the Symphony:** Heat the olive oil in a non-stick skillet over medium heat. Add the mushrooms, sautéing until golden. Introduce the spinach, wilting it to a tender melody, followed by the tomatoes, cooking until warm.
3. **Let It Flow:** Pour the egg mixture over the veggies in the skillet, tilting to ensure an even spread. Cook undisturbed, letting the eggs set gently firm, capturing the essence of the veggies.
4. **Fold and Serve:** Once the surface softly sets, fold the omelet in half, wrapping the veggie bounty inside. Slide onto a plate, a masterpiece of morning nourishment.

Summary:

Start your day with our **Veggie Omelette,** a celebration of fresh, vibrant flavors and textures. This dish isn't just breakfast; it's a journey through a garden of delight wrapped in the comfort of eggs. It's ready to energize your day with wholesomeness and joy.

EGG MUFFINS WITH FETA AND SPINACH

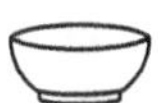

Prep Time: 10 min

Cook Time: 20 min

Serves: 6

Ingredients

- 6 large eggs (the morning's main characters)
- 1 cup spinach, chopped (a green, leafy embrace)
- 1/2 cup feta cheese, crumbled (the tangy treasure)
- 1/2 cup bell peppers, diced (a confetti of colors)
- Salt and pepper, to taste (the flavor enhancers)
- A drizzle of olive oil (for the muffin pan)

Nutritional Information:

Per serving: Estimated values: 150 calories, 10g protein, 3g carbohydrates, 10g fat, 1g fiber, 185mg cholesterol, 320mg sodium, 200mg potassium.

Directions

1. **Warm up and set the stage:** Preheat your oven to 350°F. Gently grease a muffin tin with olive oil to prevent any sticking.
2. **Whisk and Mix:** In a large bowl, crack the eggs and give them a good whisk, adding a pinch of salt and pepper. Mix in the chopped spinach, crumbled feta, and diced bell peppers until everything is lovingly combined.
3. **Pour and Bake:** Evenly distribute the egg mixture into the prepared muffin tin. Slide it into the oven and bake until the muffins are firm and golden about 20 minutes.
4. **Serve with Joy:** Let the muffins cool for a few minutes before gently lifting them from the tin. Serve warm little bundles of joy, perhaps with your favorite morning toast or fresh fruit.

Summary:

Experience a bite of morning magic with our **Egg Muffins with Feta and Spinach**. Each muffin is a mini celebration, bursting with the goodness of eggs, the richness of feta, and the freshness of spinach and bell peppers. They're not just breakfast; they're little rays of sunshine, ready to brighten your day.

BERRY YOGURT PARFAIT

Ingredients

- 2 cups Greek yogurt (a creamy dream)
- 1 cup mixed berries (a sweet whisper of nature)
- 1 cup granola (the crunch in the symphony)
- Optional: honey or maple syrup for drizzling (the golden touch)

Nutritional Information: Per serving: Estimated values: 250 calories, 12g protein, 35g carbohydrates, 8g fat, 5g fiber, 10mg cholesterol, 65mg sodium, and 200mg potassium.

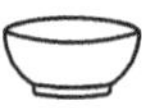  

Prep Time: 10 min   Cook Time: 0 min   Serves: 4

Directions

1. **A layer of Love:** Begin with a dollop of Greek yogurt at the bottom of four glasses or jars, creating a cloud-like foundation. For an extra touch of elegance, use a piping bag to create a neat, even layer.
2. **Berry Bliss:** Scatter a layer of mixed berries over the yogurt, like jewels upon a crown.
3. **Crunchy Crescendo:** Sprinkle granola on top of the berries, adding texture and depth to your creation.
4. **Repeat and Drizzle:** Repeat the layers until the glasses are filled to the brim. If desired, drizzle a touch of honey or maple syrup over the top for a kiss of sweetness.

Summary:

The **Berry Yogurt Parfait** is not just a delicious treat but also a nutritious start to your day as a melody of textures and tastes celebrating simple ingredients coming together in perfect harmony. Start your day on a note of pure joy.

TROPICAL YOGURT PARFAIT

Ingredients

- 2 cups coconut yogurt (a creamy, tropical embrace)
- 1 cup mango, diced (sunshine in a bite)
- 1 cup pineapple, diced (a splash of joy)
- 1/4 cup toasted coconut flakes (a whisper of island dreams)

Nutritional Information: Per serving: Estimated values: 230 calories, 5g protein, 36g carbohydrates, 7g fat, 3g fiber, 0mg cholesterol, 30mg sodium, 400mg potassium.

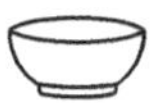  

Prep Time: 10 min   Cook Time: 0 min   Serves: 4

Directions

1. **Begin with Bliss:** Spoon a generous layer of coconut yogurt into the bottom of four glasses, laying the foundation for a tropical escape.
2. **Sun-Kissed Layers:** Add a layer of diced mango over the yogurt, followed by a layer of pineapple, painting each glass with vibrant colors and tropical flavors.
3. **Island Crunch:** Sprinkle a layer of toasted coconut flakes on top, adding texture and deepening the tropical narrative.
4. **Repeat the Retreat:** Layering the yogurt, mango, pineapple, and coconut until the glasses are full, finishing with a sprinkle of coconut flakes as a final nod to the islands.

Summary:

Dive into the **Tropical Yogurt Parfait**, a dish that's not just breakfast but a passport to paradise. It's more than a meal; it's a moment of escape, a brief vacation in a glass, inviting you to savor the sweetness of life with every spoonful.

Apple Pie Parfait

Ingredients

- 1 cup Greek yogurt (a creamy canvas)
- 2 large apples, peeled and diced (the taste of autumn)
- 1 teaspoon ground cinnamon (a sprinkle of nostalgia)
- 1 tablespoon butter (for richness)
- 1 cup granola (the crunch of comfort)
- Optional: honey or maple syrup for drizzling (the sweetness of memories)

Nutritional Information: Per serving: Estimated values: 280 calories are 12g protein, 40g carbohydrates, 8g fat, 4g fiber, 15mg cholesterol, 60mg sodium, and 300mg potassium.

-

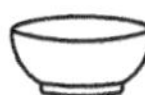  

Prep Time: 15 min   Cook Time: 10 min   Serves: 4

Directions

1. **Stew with Love:** In a pan, melt the butter over medium heat. Add the diced apples and cinnamon, stirring until the apples are soft and caramelized, about 10 minutes. Let this sweet concoction cool slightly.
2. **Layer of Dreams:** Spoon a layer of Greek yogurt into each glass, smooth and serene, waiting for its complement.
3. **Autumn Embrace:** Add a layer of cinnamon-kissed apples over the yogurt, each piece a tender reminder of cozy days.
4. **Crunchy Crescendo:** Top with a generous layer of granola, introducing a satisfying texture that sings against the softness of the yogurt and apples.

Summary:

The **Apple Pie Parfait** is more than a dish; it's a journey back to the heartwarming moments of autumn, captured in layers of lush yogurt, spiced apples, and the homey crunch of granola. Each spoonful is a comforting embrace, a blend of flavors and textures that evoke the simple pleasures of a homemade apple pie, served with a twist of health and happiness. It's a tribute to the days of fall, an invitation to savor the sweet, spice-kissed essence of the season anytime, anywhere.

Peanut Butter Chocolate Parfait

Ingredients

- 2 cups Greek yogurt (a velvety embrace)
- 4 tablespoons peanut butter (a nutty whisper)
- 2 tablespoons cocoa powder (a chocolate dream)
- 2 bananas, sliced (sweet slices of joy)
- For an added touch of sweetness, consider a delicate drizzle of honey or maple syrup (a hint of sweetness)

Nutritional Information: Per serving: Estimated values: 320 calories, 15g protein, 38g carbohydrates, 14g fat, 5g fiber, 10mg cholesterol, 150mg sodium, 400mg potassium.

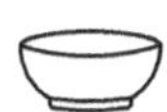  

Prep Time: 10 min   Cook Time: 0 min   Serves: 4

Directions

1. **Mix with Love:** Blend the Greek yogurt with cocoa powder in a bowl until you achieve a smooth, chocolatey foundation. If you like a touch of sweetness, incorporate a touch of maple syrup or honey, whisking gently to introduce a subtle, sweet undertone for a slight hint of sweetness for a subtle hint of sweetness.
2. **Layer of Happiness**: Spoon a layer of the chocolate yogurt mixture into each serving glass, laying the groundwork for a delicious journey.
3. **Nutty Heart:** Spread peanut butter gently over the yogurt to create a seamless blend of flavors.
4. **Joyful Topping:** Arrange banana slices on the peanut butter, adding a natural sweetness and a bright contrast to the rich layers beneath

Summary:

The **Peanut Butter Chocolate Parfait** is not just a dessert; it's a celebration in a glass, where every layer is an invitation to treat yourself to the irresistible allure of peanut butter and chocolate, indulging in their comforting embrace, balanced with the freshness of bananas. This parfait is a harmonious blend of textures and tastes, a reminder of simple pleasures and moments of bliss.

CHIA SEED PUDDING PARFAIT

Ingredients

- 1/2 cup chia seeds (little specks of magic)
- 2 cups almond milk (the Velvet River)
- 1 tablespoon of honey or maple syrup (the sweet whisper)
- 1 teaspoon vanilla extract (a hint of mystery)
- 1 cup mixed berries (the colorful laughter of nature)
- 1/4 cup almond slivers (the crunchy applause)

Nutritional Information:
Per serving: Estimated values: 250 calories, 8g protein, 24g carbohydrates, 15g fat, 10g fiber, 0mg cholesterol, 120mg sodium, 350mg potassium.

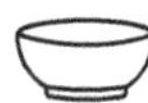  

Prep Time: 15 min (plus overnight soaking) Cook Time: 0 min Serves: 4

Directions

1. **Nighttime Whisper:** In a large bowl, mix the chia seeds with almond milk, honey (or maple syrup), and vanilla extract. Stir gently until well combined, letting each seed soak in the melody of flavors.
2. **Dream in Layers:** Cover and let the mixture rest in the refrigerator overnight. The chia seeds will swell, creating a pudding that holds the night's dreams and the promise of the morning.
3. **Morning Assembly:** Once the chia pudding has been set, take four glasses and layer the pudding with mixed berries, creating a tapestry of colors and textures. Each layer is a stroke of flavor, a blend of sweet and tart, soft and crunchy.
4. **Final Flourish:** Sprinkle almond slivers on top for a final touch of crunch, a nod to the morning sun that shines bright and promises a day full of possibilities.

Summary:

The **Chia Seed Pudding Parfait** is not just a dish; it's a journey from night to day, a blend of textures and flavors that speaks of comfort, nourishment, and the simple joys of eating. Each spoonful is a discovery, a moment to savor, bringing together the earthy sweetness of chia, the freshness of berries, and the satisfying crunch of almonds. It's a breakfast, a snack, a moment of peace—a reminder that the best things in life are often layered and waiting to be explored.

QUINOA BREAKFAST BOWL

Ingredients

- 1 cup quinoa (the tiny but mighty heart of the dish)
- 2 cups water (for cooking the quinoa)
- 1 tablespoon of olive oil (a splash of silkiness)
- 2 cups kale, chopped (a green hug in every bite)
- 1 cup cherry tomatoes, halved (little bursts of joy)
- 4 large eggs (the morning's sun)
- Salt and pepper, to taste (the flavor whisperers)

Nutritional Information:
Per serving: Estimated values: 320 calories: 14g protein, 38g carbohydrates, 12g fat, 6g fiber, 186mg cholesterol, 200mg sodium, and 400mg potassium

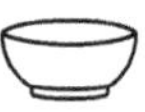  

Prep Time: 10 min Cook Time: 20 min Serves: 4

Directions

1. **Quinoa's Journey:** Rinse the quinoa under cold water, then combine it with water in a saucepan. Bring to a boil, then reduce to a simmer, cover, and let it cook until fluffy and tender, about 15 minutes.
2. **Green Embrace:** Heat olive oil over medium heat while the quinoa cooks. Add the kale, season with some salt and pepper, and sauté until just wilted and vibrant, for about 5 minutes. Toss in the cherry tomatoes for the last minute to warm them through.
3. **Egg's Sunshine:** Softly boil the eggs by gently placing them in boiling water for 6-7 minutes for that perfectly runny yolk, then plunge them into cold water to stop the cooking process.
4. **Assemble with Love:** Scoop the quinoa into bowls, top with the sautéed kale and tomatoes, and carefully peel and place an egg on each. Season with a final pinch of Salt and pepper.

Summary:

Welcome to the **Quinoa Breakfast Bowl**, where each ingredient is a note in a symphony of flavors and textures. This dish isn't just breakfast; it's a morning ritual that nourishes your body, delights your taste buds, and sets the tone for the day ahead. With every forkful, experience the wholesome nuttiness of quinoa, the tender embrace of kale, the joyful pop of cherry tomatoes, and the creamy richness of a perfectly soft-boiled egg. It's a bowl full of health, happiness, and a promise of a good day.

Sweet Potato Hash

Ingredients

- 2 large sweet potatoes, peeled and diced (sunshine cubes)
- 1 tablespoon olive oil (liquid gold)
- 1 medium onion, diced (the flavor foundation)
- 1 bell pepper, diced (colorful crunch)
- 4 large eggs (morning's glory)
- Salt and pepper, to taste (the taste enhancers)
- Optional: fresh herbs for garnish (a green sprinkle of joy)

Nutritional Information:
Per serving: Estimated values: 300 calories, 12g protein, 35g carbohydrates, 12g fat, 6g fiber, 185mg cholesterol, 220mg sodium, 800mg potassium

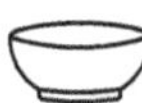  

Prep Time: 15 min   Cook Time: 20 min   Serves: 4

Directions

1. **Roast the Sunshine:** Heat the olive oil over medium heat in a large skillet. Toss in the sweet potatoes and let them sizzle and soften, turning golden and slightly crispy for about 10 minutes.
2. **Add Color and Crunch:** Stir in the onion and bell pepper, seasoning with a pinch of Salt and pepper. Cook until the onions are translucent, and peppers are tender, adding a symphony of flavors to the sweet potatoes, about 5 minutes more.
3. **Scramble the Dawn:** In a separate pan, gently scramble the eggs to your liking, seasoning them with Salt and pepper. The eggs should be soft and creamy, perfecting the hash.
4. **Morning Assembly:** Serve the sweet potato hash warm, topped with the softly scrambled eggs and a sprinkle of fresh herbs if desired.

Summary:

Step into the morning light with our **Sweet Potato Hash**, a dish that brings together the heartiness of sweet potatoes with the tender bite of onions and bell peppers, all crowned with the comfort of scrambled eggs. It isn't just a meal; it's a warm embrace to start your day, a plate full of colors, textures, and flavors that whisper of comfort, care, and the simple joy of a morning well-begun.

Avocado Chickpea Toast

Ingredients

- 1 can (15 oz) chickpeas, drained and rinsed (the heart of the dish)
- 1 ripe avocado (the creamy dream)
- 4 slices of whole-grain bread (the sturdy base)
- Salt and pepper, to taste (the flavor dancers)
- A handful of sprouts (the fresh finish)

Nutritional Information:
Per serving: Estimated values: 280 calories, 10g protein, 38g carbohydrates, 12g fat, 9g fiber, 0mg cholesterol, 300mg sodium, and 400mg potassium.

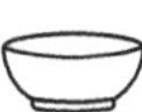  

Prep Time: 10 min   Cook Time: 0 min   Serves: 4

Directions

1. **Mash and Mix:** Combine chickpeas and avocado in a bowl. Mash them with a fork or potato masher until you have a beautifully textured spread. Season with Salt and pepper to your taste.
2. **Toast to Perfection:** Lightly toast the whole-grain bread slices to your liking, giving them a warm, crispy edge that will hold up to the spread.
3. **Spread the Joy:** Generously spread the chickpea and avocado mixture over each slice of toast, creating a thick layer of creamy goodness.
4. **Top with Life:** Sprinkle a handful of sprouts over the top of each toast, adding a burst of freshness and a hint of crunch.

Summary:

Embark on a journey of flavor and nourishment with **Avocado Chickpea Toast**, a simple yet profoundly satisfying dish that marries the rich, buttery texture of avocado with the hearty, earthy essence of chickpeas, all resting atop a slice of crunchy, wholesome bread. Each mouthful adorned with a sprinkle of sprouts celebrates vitality and well-being, inviting a pause to relish nature's vibrant, unadulterated flavors.

Zucchini Pancakes

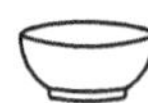

Ingredients

- 2 medium zucchinis, shredded (the green stars)
- 2 large eggs (the binders of joy)
- 1/2 cup all-purpose flour (the subtle backbone)
- 1/4 teaspoon salt (the flavor enhancer)
- 1/4 teaspoon pepper (a gentle kick)
- 2 tablespoons olive oil (for golden moments)
- 1/2 cup Greek yogurt (the creamy dream)
- Fresh herbs (like dill or parsley for a green flourish)

Nutritional Information: Per serving: Estimated values: 220 calories, 8g protein, 18g carbohydrates, 12g fat, 2g fiber, 105mg cholesterol, 200mg sodium, and 300mg potassium.

Prep Time: 15 min

Cook Time: 10 min

Serves: 4

Directions

1. **Combine with Care:** In a bowl, mix the shredded zucchini, eggs, flour, Salt, and pepper until you have a harmonious batter ready to transform.
2. **Pan-Fry to Perfection:** Heat a swirl of olive oil in a skillet over medium heat. Dollop the zucchini mixture into the pan, flattening slightly. Cook until each side is a golden tribute to the sun, about 4-5 minutes per side.
3. **Serve with Love:** Plate your zucchini pancakes warm, dolloping Greek yogurt on top for a creamy contrast, and sprinkle with fresh herbs to nod to the garden's bounty.
4. **Savor the Moment:** Pause to admire your creation before diving into the flavors, textures, and warmth that await.

Summary:

Embarking on a culinary adventure with **Zucchini Pancakes**, a dish that wraps the freshness of the garden in a warm, inviting embrace. These pancakes are not just a meal; they celebrate simplicity and nourishment. Each bite is a reminder of the joy found in wholesome ingredients, brought together with care and served with love. It's a dish that comforts satisfies, and inspires, making any meal a moment to cherish.

Breakfast Salad

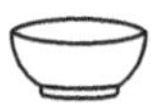

Ingredients

- 4 cups mixed greens (a bed of morning dew)
- 1 cup cooked quinoa (the sunrise grains)
- 1 ripe avocado, sliced (the creamy dream)

For the vinaigrette:

- 2 tablespoons olive oil (the liquid gold)
- 1 tablespoon of lemon juice (a zesty awakening)
- Salt and pepper, to taste (the flavor dance)
- 4 large eggs (the morning suns)

Prep Time: 15 min

Cook Time: 10 min

Serves: 4

Directions

1. **Dress in Joy:** In a small bowl, whisk together the olive oil, lemon juice, Salt, and pepper until the vinaigrette is born, bright and lively.
2. **Toss with Care:** In a large bowl, gently toss the mixed greens and cooked quinoa with the lemon vinaigrette, coating each leaf and grain in a layer of zestful love.
3. **Poach with Precision:** Bring a pot of water to a gentle simmer. Crack each egg into the water and poach to your liking, about 3-4 minutes for runny yolks, the essence of a gentle sunrise.
4. **Assemble with Heart:** Divide the salad among plates, top each with slices of avocado and a poached egg, tender and warm.

Nutritional Information: Per serving: 320 calories, 14g protein, 24g carbohydrates, 20g fat, 7g fiber, 186mg cholesterol, 210mg sodium, and 450mg potassium.

Summary:

Step into the light of the **Breakfast Salad,** where morning greens meet the golden touch of the sun in the form of a poached egg. It transcends mere sustenance, an awakening, a celebration of freshness and vitality that promises to start your day with pure joy and satisfaction. It's a salad that doesn't whisper but sings, heralding a day filled with promise and light.

Grilled Vegetable Quinoa Bowl

Ingredients

- 1 cup quinoa (the wholesome base)
- 2 cups water (for cooking quinoa)
- 1 zucchini, sliced into rounds (the summer favorite)
- 1 red bell pepper, sliced into strips (the sweet crunch)
- 1 yellow bell pepper, sliced into strips (the sunny lift)
- 1 small eggplant, sliced into rounds (the hearty touch)
- 1 red onion, cut into wedges (the bold flavor)
- 2 tablespoons olive oil (
- Salt and pepper, to taste
- 1/4 cup balsamic reduction
- Fresh basil leaves for garnish

Nutritional Information:

Per serving: Estimated values: 320 calories, 10g protein, 55g carbohydrates, 9g fat, 8g fiber, 0mg cholesterol, 320mg sodium, 350mg potassium.

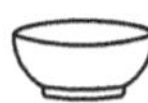  

Prep Time: 20 min | Cook Time: 30 min | Serves: 4

Directions

1. **Preparing Quinoa:** Start by washing the quinoa under cold water thoroughly. In a pot, bring 2 cups of water to a boil. Please put on the quinoa, turn down the heat to low, cover, and let it simmer for about 15 minutes or until the water is completely absorbed. Once finished, fluff the quinoa with a fork and let it cool.
2. **Prep and Grill Vegetables:** Preheat the grill to medium-high. Toss zucchini, bell peppers, eggplant, and red onion with olive oil, salt, and pepper. Grill vegetables until charred and tender, about 5-7 minutes per side, turning once. The grilling brings out their natural sweetness and adds a smoky depth.
3. **Assemble Bowls:** Divide the cooked quinoa among four bowls. Arrange the grilled vegetables beautifully on top of the quinoa, creating a vibrant mosaic of colors and textures.
4. **Drizzle and Garnish:** Drizzle each bowl with balsamic reduction for a tangy sweetness that ties all the flavors together. Garnish with fresh basil leaves to add freshness and a hint of elegance.
5. **Serve and Enjoy:** Serve the bowls immediately, offering a nourishing, flavorful meal that's as pleasing to the eyes as it is to the palate.

Summary:

The **Grilled Vegetable Quinoa Bowl** isn't just food; it's a feast of flavors and a tribute to healthy eating. The colorful array of vegetables, each grilled to perfection, sits atop a bed of fluffy, nutty quinoa, creating a dish that's as nutritious as it is delicious.

Vegetarian Lettuce Wraps Recipe

Ingredients

- 8 large lettuce leaves (the crisp holders)
- 1 tablespoon olive oil (for sautéing)
- 1 block (fourteen ounces) of firm tofu, crumbled (the main protein)
- 1 cup of mushrooms, finely chopped (for umami taste)
- 1-half cup water chestnuts, diced (for crunch)
- 2 green onions, thinly sliced (for a sharp flavor)
- 2 cloves garlic, minced (to enhance taste)
- 1 tablespoon of ginger, minced (for a zesty flavor)
- 3 tablespoons hoisin sauce (for a sweet and tangy coating)
- 1 tablespoon soy sauce (for depth of flavor)
- 1 teaspoon of sesame oil
- **Optional:** Sriracha or chili

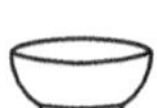  

Prep Time: 15 min | Cook Time: 10 min | Serves: 4

Directions

1. **Prepare Tofu Mixture:** Heat olive oil over medium heat in a skillet. Add the minced garlic and ginger to the pan, cooking until fragrant. Add the crumbled tofu and chopped mushrooms, sautéing until the mushrooms are tender and the tofu has browned about five to seven minutes.
2. **Add Flavors:** Mix in diced water chestnuts and sliced green onions. Pour in hoisin sauce and soy sauce, cooking for two to three minutes until well mixed and heated. Finish by drizzling with sesame oil to layer the flavors.
3. **Assemble Wraps:** Distribute the tofu mixture among the lettuce leaves, centering the filling. If desired, add Sriracha or chili flakes for a spicy kick.
4. **Serve Fresh:** Fold the lettuce around the filling and serve promptly to preserve the lettuce's freshness and crispness.

Nutritional Information:

Per serving: Estimated values: 180 calories, 12 grams protein, 15 grams carbohydrates, 9 grams fat, 4 grams fiber, 0 milligrams cholesterol, 500 milligrams sodium, 300 milligrams potassium

Summary:

These **Vegetarian Lettuce Wraps** are a lively mix of textures and flavors, offering a refreshing and satisfying meal. The hearty tofu and mushroom blend, enriched with the crunch of water chestnuts and the zest of hoisin sauce, creates a fulfilling and delicious vegetarian option.

ALMOND BUTTER BANANA WRAPS

Ingredients

- 4 whole-grain wraps (the cozy blanket)
- 1/2 cup almond butter (the nutty embrace)
- 2 bananas, sliced (sweet whispers of joy)
- Optional: A sprinkle of cinnamon or drizzle of honey (for that extra sparkle)

Nutritional Information: Per serving: Estimated values: 310 calories, 8g protein, 40g carbohydrates, 14g fat, 6g fiber, 0mg cholesterol, 200mg sodium, and 300mg potassium.

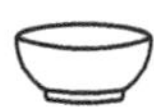  

Prep Time: 5 min   Cook Time: 0 min   Serves: 4

Directions

1. **Lay the Foundation:** Place the whole grain wraps on a flat surface, each ready to cradle the filling with open arms.
2. **Spread the Love:** Evenly spread the almond butter over each wrap, creating a rich, creamy layer that will last through the morning hustle.
3. **Add the Joy:** Arrange banana slices over the almond butter, dotting each wrap with sweet, mellow flavors and a smile in every bite.
4. **Roll into Delight:** Carefully roll each wrap carefully and fold in the edges to secure the precious contents. Slice in half if desired, revealing the beautiful layers of happiness within.

Summary:

Embrace the morning with **Almond Butter Banana Wraps**, a simple yet profoundly delightful way to start your day. It's a recipe that wraps comfort, joy, and nourishment into a convenient, hand-held treasure. Each bite melds the hearty goodness of whole grains with the rich, nutty layers of almond butter and the natural sweetness of bananas. Perfect for those mornings when time is fleeting, but the need for something warm, comforting, and energizing is paramount.

VEGGIE BREAKFAST BURRITOS

Ingredients

- 4 whole-grain tortillas (the warm embrace)
- 6 large eggs, scrambled (the morning's golden glow)
- 1 cup black beans, rinsed and drained (little pearls of nourishment)
- 1 cup salsa (a vibrant dance of tomatoes and spices)
- 1 tablespoon of olive oil (for cooking the eggs)
- Salt and pepper, to taste (the flavor harmonizers)
- Optional toppings: avocado slices, shredded cheese, or a dollop of Greek yogurt (for extra joy)

Nutritional Information: Per serving: Estimated values: 350 calories, 20g protein, 35g carbohydrates, 15g fat, 8g fiber, 280mg cholesterol, 500mg sodium, and 400mg potassium.

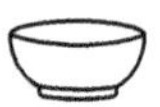  

Prep Time: 15 min   Cook Time: 10 min   Serves: 4

Directions

1. **Scramble with Love:** Heat the olive oil in a skillet over medium heat. Whisk the eggs with a pinch of Salt and pepper, and gently pour them into the skillet.
2. **Warmth and Wrap:** Warm the whole-grain tortillas in a separate pan or the microwave just until they're pliable and warm, ready to hold the treasures you'll wrap inside.
3. **Build the Dream:** Lay out the warm tortillas and evenly distribute the scrambled eggs across each. Top with black beans and a generous spoonful of salsa, inviting a burst of flavors and colors.
4. **Roll into Morning:** Carefully roll up each tortilla, tucking in the sides to enclose the filling snugly. Add any optional toppings like avocado, cheese, or a dollop of Greek yogurt for a creamy finish.

Summary:

Welcome to **Veggie Breakfast Burritos**, a heartwarming ensemble of whole-grain tortillas filled with the softest scrambled eggs, hearty black beans, and spirited salsa. This dish is a morning symphony, a fusion of textures and tastes that wraps you in comfort and readiness for the day ahead. It's not just breakfast; it's a promise of a beautiful day, each bite a step filled with energy, nutrition, and the simple pleasure of good food. Here's to mornings that taste like joy and feel like an embrace.

APPLE SANDWICHES

Ingredients

- 2 large apples, cored and sliced into rounds (nature's sweet plates)
- 1/2 cup almond butter (the creamy heart)
- 1/4 cup granola (the crunch of joy)
- A sprinkle of cinnamon (a whisper of warmth)

Nutritional Information: Per serving: Estimated values: 220 calories, 4g protein, 24g carbohydrates, 12g fat, 5g fiber, 0mg cholesterol, 0mg sodium, and 200mg potassium.

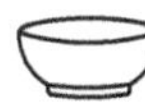

Prep Time: 5 min   Cook Time: 0 min   Serves: 4

Directions

1. **Prepare the Canvas:** Core and slice the apples into round, sturdy slices, each one a perfect circle of crispness and sweetness.
2. **Spread the Love:** On half of the apple slices, spread a generous layer of almond butter, covering the surface with a creamy, nutty blanket.
3. **Add the Sparkle:** Sprinkle granola over the almond butter, adding a delightful crunch and contrast to the softness beneath. A dash of cinnamon adds a final touch of spice, like a cozy hug.
4. **Sandwich the Magic:** Top each almond butter and granola-covered apple slice with another apple slice, pressing gently to secure the filling. Each sandwich is a bite of harmony, a blend of textures and tastes.

Summary:

Apple Sandwiches are a simple, whimsical creation that transforms everyday ingredients into a celebration of flavors and textures. It's a dish that invites you to play, savor, and enjoy the moment, with each bite a perfect balance of crisp apple, creamy almond butter, and crunchy granola.

BREAKFAST SMOOTHIE

Ingredients

- 2 cups fresh spinach (a green embrace)
- 1 ripe banana (sweetness in every slice)
- 2 cups almond milk (the silk of the morning)
- Ice cubes (a chill whisper)
- Optional: A tablespoon of honey or maple syrup (for those who like a sweeter sunrise)

Nutritional Information: Per serving: Estimated values: 160 calories, 3g protein, 30g carbohydrates, 3g fat, 4g fiber, 0mg cholesterol, 120mg sodium, and 400mg potassium.

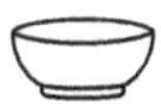

Prep Time: 5 min   Cook Time: 0 min   Serves: 2

Directions

1. **Blend the Green:** In your blender, combine the spinach and almond milk, blending until the mixture is smooth and the spinach is fully incorporated, creating a verdant liquid jewel.
2. **Sweeten the Blend:** Add the banana (and honey or maple syrup if using) to the blender, along with a few ice cubes for a refreshing chill. Blend again until smooth and creamy, like a morning cloud.
3. **Pour and Admire:** Pour the smoothie into glasses and observe the beauty of your creation, a blend of nature and nourishment.
4. **Savor the Moment:** Take a sip, and let the flavors awaken your senses, filling you with energy and a sense of well-being to carry you through the day.

Summary:

Embark on your day with the **Breakfast Smoothie,** a vitality potion combining the freshness of spinach, the sweetness of banana, and the creaminess of almond milk into a magical elixir. Treat yourself well with energy, health, and simple joy.

Ingredients

- 2 cups rolled oats (the foundation of mornings)
- 1/2 cup mixed nuts, chopped (a crunch of joy)
- 1/4 cup seeds (sunflower or pumpkin, whispers of the earth)
- 1/2 cup dried fruit (sweet memories of summer)
- 1/4 cup honey or maple syrup (nature's nectar)
- 1/2 cup almond milk (a gentle pour)
- 1 egg (the binder of dreams)
- 1 teaspoon vanilla extract (a hint of mystery)
- A pinch of Salt (the balance)

Nutritional Information: Per serving: Estimated values: 150 calories, 4g protein, 20g carbohydrates, 7g fat, 3g fiber, 18mg cholesterol, 20mg sodium, and 120mg potassium.

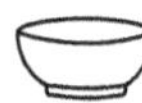

Prep Time: 15 min   Cook Time: 25min   Serves: 12 bars

Directions

1. **Mix and Mingle:** In a large bowl, combine the oats, nuts, seeds, and dried fruit. Drizzle with honey or maple syrup, add the almond milk, and crack in the egg. Pour in the vanilla extract and sprinkle with a pinch of Salt. Stir until everything is lovingly combined.
2. **Prep and Press:** Preheat your oven to 350°F (175°C). Line a baking tray with parchment paper. Pour the mixture into the tray, pressing down firmly to ensure it's compact and even.
3. **Bake and Wait:** Slide the tray into the oven and bake until the edges turn golden and the bars feel firm to the touch, about 25 minutes. The aroma will fill your kitchen, a prelude to the coming joy.
4. **Cool and Slice:** Allow the bars to cool in the tray, then transfer to a cutting board and slice into bars. Each piece is a slice of morning tranquility, ready to accompany you through the day.

Summary:

Embrace the day with **Oatmeal Breakfast Bars**, a symphony of oats, nuts, seeds, and dried fruit baked into bars of pure morning delight. Each bar is a testament to the power of simple, wholesome ingredients coming together in perfect harmony. Portable, nourishing, and endlessly customizable, these bars aren't just breakfast; they promise energy, a moment of pleasure, and a spark of joy. Perfect for busy mornings, they invite you to pause and savor, even when time is precious. Here's to starting your days on a note as sweet and satisfying as the bars themselves.

The "**Super Easy Breakfast Recipes**" chapter isn't just a collection of recipes; it's a manifesto for joyful, energetic mornings. It's about nourishing your body and spirit, even when time is a luxury. These recipes are your allies in the rush of life, ensuring that every morning is well-spent for a delicious, nutritious start.

Each recipe in this section is a love letter to the idea that breakfast can be as savory, satisfying, and exciting as any meal of the day. It's an invitation to start your mornings with intention, savoring each bite and nourishing your body and spirit.

These dishes aren't just food; they're a way to celebrate the dawn of a new day with joy, flavor, and a little adventure.

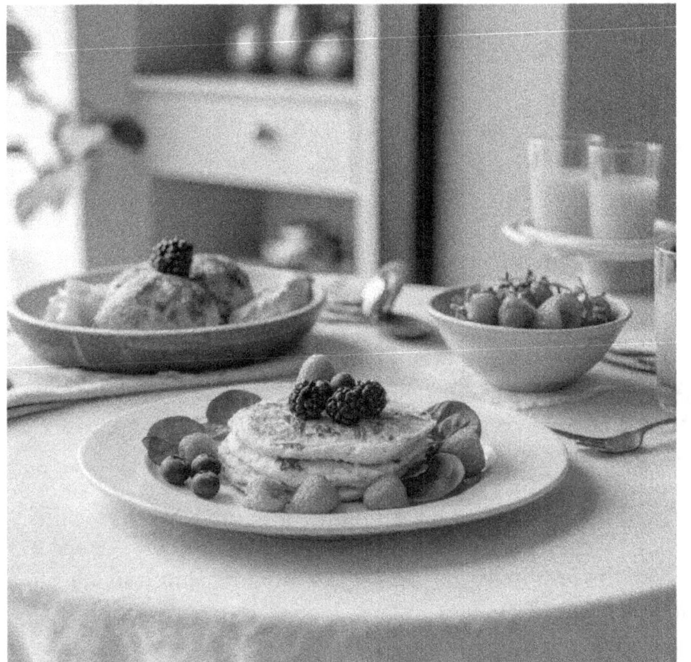

CHAPTER 4: WEEKEND BRUNCH SPECIALS

Step into the cozy, comforting world of **"Weekend Brunch Specials"** from our **"Delicious Diabetic Cookbook for Beginners,"** where each recipe celebrates leisurely mornings and the joy of eating well.

This chapter is a treasure trove of delights that marry the simplicity of ingredients with the elegance of flavors, all while keeping your health in the forefront.

This chapter isn't just a collection of recipes; it's an invitation to create moments of connection, joy, and wellness.

Whether cooking for yourself or sharing with loved ones, these **"Weekend Brunch Specials"** promise to make your mornings memorable. They blend the care for diabetic health with the unabashed pleasure of delicious, heartwarming food.

Here's to brunches that feel like a hug and weekends that taste like happiness.

SWEET POTATO WAFFLES

Ingredients

- 2 cups rolled oats (the foundation of mornings)
- 1/2 cup mixed nuts, chopped (a crunch of joy)
- 1/4 cup seeds (sunflower or pumpkin, whispers of the earth)
- 1/2 cup dried fruit (sweet memories of summer)
- 1/4 cup honey or maple syrup (nature's nectar)
- 1/2 cup almond milk (a gentle pour)
- 1 egg (the binder of dreams)
- 1 teaspoon vanilla extract (a hint of mystery)
- A pinch of Salt (the balance)

Nutritional Information:
Per serving: Estimated values: 150 calories, 4g protein, 20g carbohydrates, 7g fat, 3g fiber, 18mg cholesterol, 20mg sodium, and 120mg potassium.

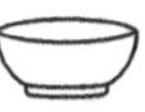 Prep Time: 15 min

 Cook Time: 25min

 Serves: 12 bars

Directions

5. **Mix and Mingle:** In a large bowl, combine the oats, nuts, seeds, and dried fruit. Drizzle with honey or maple syrup, add the almond milk, and crack in the egg. Pour in the vanilla extract and sprinkle with a pinch of Salt. Stir until everything is lovingly combined.
6. **Prep and Press:** Preheat your oven to 350°F (175°C). Line a baking tray with parchment paper. Pour the mixture into the tray, pressing down firmly to ensure it's compact and even.
7. **Bake and Wait:** Slide the tray into the oven and bake until the edges turn golden and the bars feel firm to the touch, about 25 minutes. The aroma will fill your kitchen, a prelude to the coming joy.
8. **Cool and Slice:** Allow the bars to cool in the tray, then transfer to a cutting board and slice into bars. Each piece is a slice of morning tranquility, ready to accompany you through the day.

Summary:

Embrace the day with **Oatmeal Breakfast Bars**, a symphony of oats, nuts, seeds, and dried fruit baked into bars of pure morning delight. Each bar is a testament to the power of simple, wholesome ingredients coming together in perfect harmony. Portable, nourishing, and endlessly customizable, these bars aren't just breakfast; they promise energy, a moment of pleasure, and a spark of joy. Perfect for busy mornings, they invite you to pause and savor, even when time is precious. Here's to starting your days on a note as sweet and satisfying as the bars themselves.

BAKED AVOCADO EGGS

Ingredients

- 2 ripe avocados (the green embrace)
- 4 large eggs (the morning's promise)
- Salt and pepper, to taste (the simple seasonings)
- Optional: fresh herbs, like chives or parsley, for garnish (a sprinkle of joy)

Nutritional Information: Per serving: Estimated values: 220 calories, 8g protein, 8g carbohydrates, 18g fat, 7g fiber, 185mg cholesterol, 120mg sodium, and 500mg potassium.

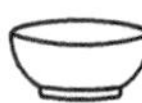  

Prep Time: 5 min   Cook Time: 15min   Serves: 4

Directions

1. **Preheat and Prepare:** Warm your oven to 425°F (220°C), and halve the avocados, removing the pit to create a cozy nest for the eggs.
2. **Nestle the Eggs:** Crack an egg into the center of each avocado half, treating it like a delicate secret. Season with Salt and pepper.
3. **Bake to Perfection:** Carefully place the avocado halves on a baking tray and slide them into the oven. Bake until the egg whites have solidified, but the yolks are still tender, about 15 minutes, like a gentle sunrise.
4. **Serve with Love:** Garnish with fresh herbs to add a burst of color and a touch of freshness to your beautiful creation.

Summary:

Step into a moment of morning tranquility with **Baked Avocado Eggs**, a recipe that marries the creamy, lush texture of avocado with the comforting warmth of baked eggs. This dish is a simple ode to the joys of eating well, offering a blend of flavors and textures that nourish both body and soul.

SALMON AND CREAM CHEESE BAGELS

Ingredients

- 4 whole-grain bagels (the hearty foundation)
- 4 ounces light cream cheese (the creamy embrace)
- 8 ounces smoked salmon (the star of the morning)
- 1 tablespoon capers (little bursts of flavor)
- Optional: thin slices of red onion, tomato slices, or a sprinkle of dill for garnish (layers of joy)

Nutritional Information: Per serving: Estimated values: 360 calories, 25g protein, 40g carbohydrates, 12g fat, 6g fiber, 30mg cholesterol, 620mg sodium, 300mg potassium.

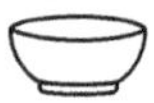  

Prep Time: 5 min   Cook Time: 0 min   Serves: 4

Directions

1. **Begin with the Base:** Slice each bagel in half and toast them to your liking, seeking that perfect golden hue and crispy edge that sings of morning readiness.
2. **Spread the Love:** Generously spread the light cream cheese on each bagel half, creating a soft, creamy layer ready to welcome the salmon with open arms.
3. **Layer the Luxe:** Carefully drape slices of smoked salmon over the cream cheese, each piece a silk of the sea, rich and inviting.
4. **Add the Sparkle:** Scatter capers over the salmon for a hint of briny brightness. If you're feeling extra, add slices of red onion, tomato, or a sprinkle of dill, each adding its whisper of flavor and freshness.

Summary:

Dive into the sumptuous world of **Salmon and Cream Cheese Bagels,** a recipe that not only transforms the simple bagel into a canvas of exquisite flavors but also provides a healthy dose of omega-3 fatty acids from the salmon and a good source of protein from the cream cheese. Here's to mornings that feel like a gentle indulgence, a plate that holds food, and a promise of a beautiful day ahead.

RICOTTA AND BERRY STUFFED FRENCH TOAST

Ingredients

- 8 slices of whole-grain bread (the sturdy vessels of joy)
- 1 cup ricotta cheese (the creamy heart)
- 1 cup mixed berries (the sweet whispers of nature)
- 2 large eggs (the golden embrace)
- 1/2 cup almond milk (the gentle mixer)
- 1 teaspoon of vanilla extract (a splash of essence)
- 2 tablespoons honey or maple syrup (the drizzle of sweetness)
- A pinch of cinnamon
- Olive oil or butter for pan-frying (the golden touch)

Nutritional Information: Per serving: Estimated values: 350 calories, 18g protein, 45g carbohydrates, 12g fat, 6g fiber, 110mg cholesterol, 320mg sodium, 250mg potassium.

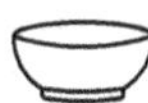  

Prep Time: 15 min   Cook Time: 10 min   Serves: 4

Directions

1. **Prep the Filling:** Gently mix the ricotta cheese with the berries, sweetening with a tablespoon of honey or maple syrup in a bowl. This mixture is your blissful filling, a creamy and sweet surprise.
2. **Ready the Bread:** Take two slices of whole-grain bread, spreading a generous layer of the ricotta and berry mixture on one slice before topping it with the other, creating a joy-filled sandwich.
3. **Whisk for Coating:** In another bowl, whisk together the eggs, almond milk, vanilla extract, and a dash of cinnamon, creating a bath of flavor for your French toast.
4. **Dip and Cook:** Heat a swipe of olive oil or a pat of butter over medium heat. Dip your stuffed bread into the egg mixture, ensuring both sides are well coated, then lay it in the pan. Cook until each side is golden brown and the filling is warmed, about 4-5 minutes per side.
5. **Serve with Love:** Serve your Ricotta and Berry Stuffed French Toast warm, drizzle with the remaining honey or maple syrup, and add some cinnamon for morning magic.

Summary:

Embark on a morning journey with the **Ricotta and Berry Stuffed French Toast.** This dish wraps the comfort of whole-grain bread around the tenderness of ricotta and the joyous burst of berries, all coming together under a golden seal of pan-fried perfection. It isn't just breakfast; it's a moment of indulgence, a symphony of care and happiness.

HUEVOS RANCHEROS

Ingredients

- 4 corn tortillas (the golden base)
- 1 cup black beans, rinsed and drained (the hearty embrace)
- 1 avocado, sliced (the creamy dream)
- 4 large eggs (the sunrise of the dish)
- For the tomato-chili sauce:
- 1 can (14 oz) diced tomatoes (the saucy heart)
- 1 small onion, diced (the flavor foundation)
- 1 clove of garlic, minced (a hint of spice)
- 1 jalapeño, deseeded and diced (the whisper of heat)
- 1 teaspoon of cumin (the earthy touch)
- Salt and pepper, to taste (the perfect seasoning)

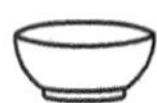  

Prep Time: 29 min   Cook Time: 15 min   Serves: 4

Directions

1. **Sauce Simmer:** In a saucepan, combine the diced tomatoes, onion, garlic, jalapeño, and cumin—season with salt and pepper to taste.
2. **Tortilla Toast:** Warm the corn tortillas in a skillet or over an open flame until they are lightly toasted and pliable, promising crunch and comfort.
3. **Eggs Delight:** In a separate pan, fry the eggs to your liking, aiming for edges crisped by the heat and yolks that still hold the morning sun.
4. **Assemble with Joy:** On each tortilla, lay a foundation of black beans and a slice of avocado, and top with a fried egg. Generously spoon the tomato-chili sauce over the egg, enveloping it in warmth and flavor.
5. **Serve and Savor:** Present your Huevos Rancheros with pride, each plate a vibrant canvas of colors, textures, and tastes.

Nutritional Information: Estimated 320 calories, 15g protein, 35g carbohydrates, 16g fat, 9g fiber, 190mg cholesterol, 410mg sodium, 700mg potassium.

Summary:

Huevos Rancheros is more than a meal; it's a morning fiesta, a vibrant celebration of life and flavor that brightens your day. Each component, from the toasted corn tortillas to the creamy avocado, the hearty black beans, and the perfectly fried eggs draped in a rich tomato-chili sauce, creates a symphony of taste that sings warmth, comfort, and joy.

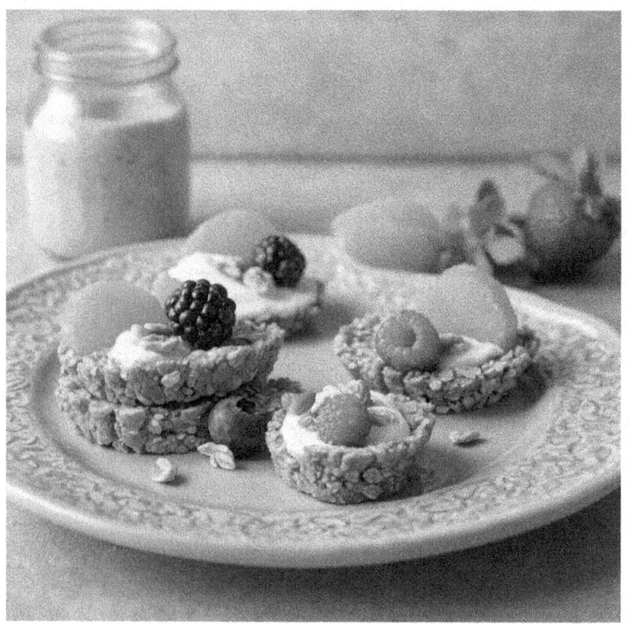

CHAPTER 5: LIGHT BITES

Dive into the "**Light Bites**" chapter of the "**Delicious Diabetic Cookbook for Beginners,**" where each recipe is a beacon of hope for mornings filled with hustle and evenings that demand simplicity. This chapter is a haven of nourishment, offering snacks and small meals that are as delightful to the palate as they benefit your health.

Fruit and Nut Breakfast Cookies break the dawn with their soft texture and the sweet, hearty mix of oats, dried fruits, and nuts. These are not just cookies; they're promises of a day filled with energy and smiles, portable delights that bring comfort and joy with every bite.

The **Cucumber Sandwiches** redefine simplicity, marrying the crisp freshness of cucumber with the creamy depth of hummus, all nestled between slices of nurturing whole-grain bread. It's a whisper of freshness, a breath of lightness that nourishes the soul and refreshes the spirit.

Carrot Cake Oatmeal Cookies are a testament to the magic of transformation, turning the humble carrot into a treat that's as wholesome as it is irresistible. With each bite, you're treated to the warmth of home-baked goodness, a gentle hug of spices, and the crunch of walnuts, reminding you that health and indulgence can walk hand in hand. **Berry Breakfast Popsicles** invites you to start your day with joy. They blend Greek yogurt and mixed berries into a frozen treat that's both refreshing and satisfying. It's a celebration of flavor, a dance of sweetness and tang that awakens the senses and cools the soul. Lastly, **Granola Cups** are a symphony of textures and tastes, a moment of delight that's as colorful as nourishing.

"**Light Bites**" is more than a chapter; it's a journey into the heart of mindful eating, a collection of recipes designed to bring lightness and joy into your meals. **Here's to the little things that make life sweet, to the bites that bring us health, happiness, and a sense of well-being.**

FRUIT AND NUT BREAKFAST COOKIES

Ingredients

- 1 cup rolled oats (the heart of the cookie)
- Use 1/2 cup whole wheat flour (for a wholesome touch)
- 1/4 cup almond milk (the gentle binder)
- 1/4 cup honey or maple syrup (a kiss of natural sweetness)
- 1/2 cup mixed dried fruit (sweet jewels)
- 1/2 cup mixed nuts, chopped (crunchy treasures)
- 1 egg (the perfect mixer)
- 1 teaspoon of vanilla extract (a dash of joy)
- 1/2 teaspoon baking powder
- Add a dash of salt

Nutritional Information: Per serving: Estimated values per cookie: 150 calories, 4g protein, 20g carbohydrates, 7g fat, 3g fiber, 15mg cholesterol, 50mg sodium, 100mg potassium.

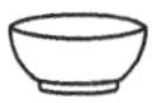  

Prep Time: 15 min   Cook Time: 12 min   Serves: 12 cookies

Directions

1. **Whisk and Blend:** In a large bowl, whisk together the oats, whole wheat flour, baking powder, and a pinch of salt. Stir in the dried fruit and nuts to coat them with the flour mixture, ensuring every bite has a bit of joy.
2. **Mix to Unite:** In another bowl, beat the egg with almond milk, honey (or maple syrup), and vanilla extract until harmoniously blended. Pour this into the dry ingredients, mixing gently until a soft, cohesive dough forms.
3. **Shape and Smile:** Preheat your oven to 350°F (175°C). Line a baking sheet with parchment paper. With joyful anticipation, shape the dough into small rounds and place them on the sheet, flattening them slightly for that perfect cookie shape.
4. **Bake to Perfection:** Slide the baking sheet into the oven and bake for about 12 minutes until the edges are golden and the centers are still dreamy. The aroma will fill your kitchen, a prelude to the delightful bites.
5. **Cool and Enjoy:** Allow the cookies to cool on the sheet for a few minutes before you transfer them to a wire rack. Now, take a moment to admire your creation.

Summary:

Each bite of **Fruit and Nut Breakfast Cookies** celebrates natural sweetness, wholesome goodness, and the delightful crunch of nuts. Perfect for busy mornings, these cookies offer a nutritious, satisfying start to your day with a bit of sweetness, and a lot of love.

CARROT CAKE OATMEAL COOKIES

Ingredients

- 1 cup rolled oats (a hug of heartiness)
- 1/2 cup whole wheat flour (the grounding touch)
- 1/2 cup grated carrots (a whisper of sweetness)
- 1/4 cup chopped walnuts (a crunch of joy)
- 1/4 cup unsweetened applesauce (nature's moistener)
- 1/4 cup raisins (little bursts of happiness)
- One egg (the golden binder)
- 1/4 cup maple syrup (a gentle kiss of sweetness)
- One teaspoon of vanilla extract
- 1/2 teaspoon baking powder
- 1/2 teaspoon cinnamon
- A pinch of salt

Nutritional Information: Per serving: 100 calories, 3g protein, 15g carbohydrates, 4g fat, 2g fiber, 18mg cholesterol, 50mg sodium, 100mg potassium.

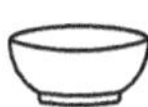  

Prep Time: 15 min   Cook Time: 12 min   Serves: 12 cookies

Directions

1. **Whisk and Wonder:** In a large bowl, whisk together the oats, whole wheat flour, baking powder, cinnamon, and a pinch of salt, setting the stage for a delightful blend.
2. **Stir and Bind:** In another bowl, stir the grated carrots, chopped walnuts, and raisins into the applesauce, egg, maple syrup, and vanilla extract, creating a harmonious mix that promises to stick together through thick and thin.
3. **Unite and Shape:** Mix the wet ingredients into the dry, stirring gently until they form a dough that hints at delicious moments ahead. With a scoop or spoon, Form the dough into rounds on a baking sheet covered with parchment paper, each cookie a testament to the beauty of baking.
4. **Bake to Perfection:** Place the tray in a 350°F (175°C) oven and bake for about 12 minutes until the edges are golden and the centers are soft yet firm, reminiscent of little suns on a cloudy day.
5. **Cool and Embrace:** Let the cookies cool for a short time on the baking sheet before moving them to a wire rack. It is in this pause, in this breath, that everything comes together in quiet anticipation.

Summary:

Carrot Cake Oatmeal Cookies are not just a treat but a journey back to the kitchen's warmth, a memory of flavors that comfort and embrace. Every bite reminds you of the simple joys that wholesome ingredients can bring. These cookies celebrate balance, where sweetness meets nourishment, and every ingredient sings harmoniously. Here's to moments savored, cherished health, and cookies that feel like home.

BERRY BREAKFAST POPSICLES

Ingredients

- 2 cups Greek yogurt (the creamy base)
- 1 cup mixed berries (fresh or frozen) (the burst of joy)
- 2 tablespoons honey or maple syrup (the whisper of sweetness)
- 1 teaspoon of vanilla extract (the hint of delight

Nutritional Information: Per serving: Estimated values per popsicle are 90 calories, 10g protein, 12g carbohydrates, 1g fat, 2g fiber, 5mg cholesterol, 30mg sodium, and 150mg potassium.

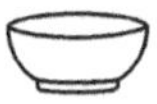  

Prep Time: 10 min (+ freezing time)   Cook Time: 0 min   Serves: 6 popsicles

Directions

1. **Blend the Joy:** In a blender, combine the Greek yogurt, mixed berries, honey (or maple syrup), and vanilla extract. Blend until the mixture is smooth, with little specks of berries creating a canvas of color and flavor.
2. **Pour the Promise:** Gently pour the mixture into popsicle molds, leaving some room at the top for expansion during freezing. If your popsicle molds come with sticks, insert them now; if not, freeze them for about an hour, then add wooden sticks.
3. **Freeze the Moment:** Put the molds in the freezer and let them freeze until solid, which should take about 4-6 hours. Leaving them overnight ensures they are thoroughly frozen and refreshingly solid for a firm, refreshing wake-up call.
4. **Release the Magic:** When ready to serve, run warm water over the outside of the molds for a few seconds to release the popsicles quickly.

Summary:

Berry Breakfast Popsicles are more than just a morning treat; they're a declaration of love for the start of each day, a refreshing embrace that cools and nourishes. Imagine greeting the morning with a popsicle; each lick is a blend of creamy Greek yogurt and the sweet, tangy burst of berries, all kissed with just a hint of honey and vanilla. It's a breakfast that breaks all the rules, inviting you to start your day with a smile and a heart full of light.

CUCUMBER SANDWICHES

Ingredients

- 8 slices of whole-grain bread (the hearty foundation)
- 1 large cucumber, thinly sliced (the crisp whisper of freshness)
- 1 cup hummus (the creamy embrace)
- Optional: Sprinkles of dill or paprika for an added touch of flavor (the little extra)

Nutritional Information: Per serving: Estimated values: 250 calories, 12g protein, 35g carbohydrates, 9g fat, 8g fiber, 0mg cholesterol, 420mg sodium, 300mg potassium.

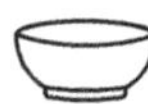  

Prep Time: 10 min · Cook Time: 0 min · Serves: 4

Directions

1. **Spread the Love:** Begin by spreading a generous layer of hummus on one side of each bread slice, creating a creamy base that's both rich and comforting.
2. **Layer with Care:** Arrange the thinly sliced cucumbers over half the bread slices, overlapping them slightly to ensure every bite includes a crunch of freshness.
3. **Season to Taste:** If you're using dill or paprika, now's the time to sprinkle it over the cucumbers, adding an extra layer of flavor that perfectly complements the crispness.
4. **Close and Serve:** Top the cucumber layers with the remaining bread slices, hummus side down. Press gently to seal the bond, then slice each sandwich in half or quarters, serving immediately to capture the essence of freshness.

Summary:

Embrace the simplicity and freshness of **Cucumber Sandwiches**, a recipe that turns everyday ingredients into a moment of pure, delightful nourishment. Ideal for a quick lunch or a refreshing snack, these sandwiches are a testament to the beauty of wholesome ingredients coming together in perfect harmony. Each bite offers a crunch of cucumber and a smooth layer of hummus, all hugged by the comforting texture of whole-grain bread. It isn't just a sandwich; it's a pause in the day, a refreshing breath that's as satisfying to the soul as it is to the palate.

GRANOLA CUPS

Ingredients

- 2 cups rolled oats (the wholesome base)
- 1/2 cup chopped nuts (a crunch of happiness)
- 1/4 cup seeds (sunflower or pumpkin, little echoes of nature)
- 1/4 cup honey or maple syrup (the sweetness of life)
- 1/4 cup melted coconut oil (the binding embrace)
- 1 teaspoon of vanilla extract (a dash of joy)
- A pinch of salt
- 1 cup Greek yogurt (the creamy dream)
- 1 cup fresh fruit (berries, kiwi, mango - the jewels of flavor.

Nutritional Information: Per serving: Estimated values per cup: 200 calories, 6g protein, 25g carbohydrates, 10g fat, 4g fiber, 5mg cholesterol, 30mg sodium, 200mg potassium.

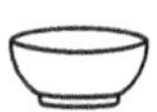  

Prep Time: 15 min · Cook Time: 15 min · Serves: 6 cups

Directions

1. **Stir and Shape:** In a large bowl, mix oats, nuts, seeds, honey (or maple syrup), melted coconut oil, vanilla extract, and a dash of salt. Stir until you lovingly coat everything. Press the mixture into muffin tins, forming little cups with your fingers or the back of a spoon, creating a nest for the yogurt.
2. **Bake to Golden:** Preheat your oven to 350°F (175°C). Bake the granola cups for about 15 minutes or until golden and hold their shape. The warmth will fill your kitchen with the promise of something delightful.
3. **Cool and Fill:** Let the granola cups cool in the pan, then carefully remove them. They're now ready to cradle the Greek yogurt, spooned gently into each cup.
4. **Crown with Color:** Top each granola cup with fresh fruit, arranging the pieces like gems on a crown. Each cup is now a treasure of flavors, textures, and joy.

Summary:

Granola Cups celebrate mornings, a crunchy, creamy, and juicy symphony that sings of new beginnings and simple pleasures. Each cup is a canvas for your favorite flavors, a masterpiece ready to be filled with the creamy delight of Greek yogurt and fresh fruit's vibrant, sweet notes. It's a breakfast that beckons you to pause, savor, and delight in each bite, offering peace and pleasure amid a busy world. Here's to starting the day with something beautiful, to mornings that taste like hope, and to the joy of creating something just for you.

Zesty Lime Shrimp Skewers

Ingredients

- 1 pound shrimp, peeled and deveined (fresh and succulent)
- Juice of 2 limes (bright and tangy)
- 1 tablespoon olive oil (for a smooth grilling experience)
- 1 clove garlic, minced (adds a burst of flavor)
- 1/2 teaspoon chili powder (for a bit of spice)
- Salt and pepper to taste (for seasoning)
- Fresh cilantro, chopped (for garnish)

Nutritional Information:

Per serving: Estimated values 180 calories, 23g protein, 3g carbohydrates, 8g fat, 1g fiber, 150mg cholesterol, 200mg sodium, 300mg potassium.

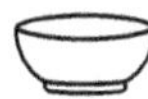  

Prep Time: 15 min   Cook Time: 10 min   Serves: 4

Directions

1. **Marinate:** Combine lime juice, olive oil, minced garlic, chili powder, salt, and pepper in a bowl. Add shrimp and toss to coat. Refrigerate for at least 30 minutes to marinate.
2. **Skewer:** Thread the marinated shrimp onto skewers.
3. **Grill:** Heat a grill or grill pan over medium heat. Grill the skewers for 2-3 minutes on each side until the shrimp turn opaque and develop a slight char.
4. **Garnish and Serve:** Sprinkle with fresh cilantro and serve immediately.

Summary:

Zesty Lime Shrimp Skewers offer a fresh, flavorful, and light option, perfect for a quick snack or meal. The tangy lime and spicy chili contrast with the succulent shrimp, making this dish a delightful treat.

Sweet Pepper and Hummus Dip

Ingredients

- 1 cup hummus (creamy and rich)
- 1 cup sweet bell peppers, diced (colorful and crunchy)
- 2 tablespoons olive oil (adds a silky texture)
- 1 tablespoon lemon juice (for a fresh zing)
- Salt and pepper to taste (for seasoning)
- A sprinkle of paprika (for a smoky hint)

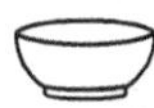  

Prep Time: 10 min   Cook Time: 0 min   Serves: 4

Directions

1. **Combine:** In a serving bowl, mix the hummus with diced sweet peppers, olive oil, and lemon juice—season with salt and pepper.
2. **Garnish:** Sprinkle paprika over the top for a touch of smokiness.
3. **Serve:** Offer this dip with fresh vegetables or whole-grain crackers for dipping.

Nutritional Information: Per serving: Estimated values: 150 calories, 4g protein, 8g carbohydrates, 12g fat, 3g fiber, 0mg cholesterol, 300mg sodium, 200mg potassium

Summary:

Sweet Pepper and Hummus Dip is an inviting, colorful snack that combines the smooth richness of hummus with the crisp sweetness of bell peppers. This recipe is an easy, quick option for anyone looking for a healthy snack that doesn't compromise flavor.

"Light Bites" isn't just a chapter; it's a journey into the heart of wholesome, joyful eating. It's about starting your day with a burst of energy or finding that perfect, satisfying snack that doesn't just feed your body but also nourishes your soul. Here's to embracing the beauty in every bite, discovering new favorites, and the little moments of happiness that homemade treats can bring into our lives.

Let these recipes remind you that every meal is an opportunity to treat yourself well, with love, care, and creativity.

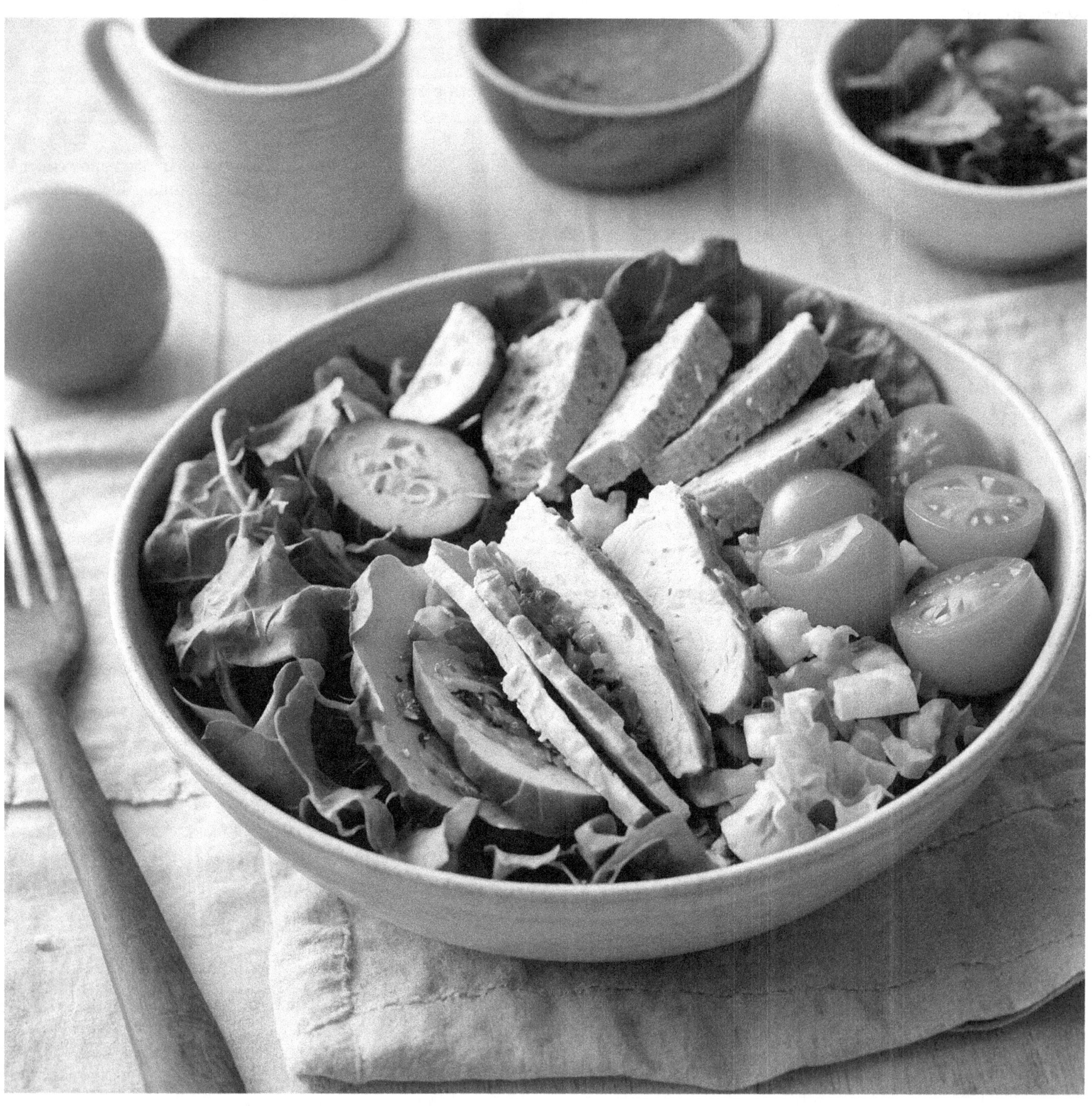

Tasty lunch ideas for home, work, or on the go: wraps, salads, and satisfying soups.

Embark on a culinary journey with **"Lunch Made Simple,"** a cherished chapter from the **"Delicious Diabetic Cookbook for Beginners."** This segment is a lovingly curated collection of lunch ideas that promise simplicity without compromising flavor or nutritional value. Designed with busy lives in mind, these recipes are a delight, whether dining at home, packing a lunch for work, or needing something wholesome.

"Lunch Made Simple" isn't just about feeding your body; it's about enriching your day with joy and satisfaction through good food. It's an invitation to transform your lunchtime routine into an opportunity for nourishment, exploration, and, perhaps most importantly, a little delight amid a busy day. And the best part? These recipes are straightforward, even for those with the busiest schedules.

Each recipe is more than just a meal; it's a small celebration of the possible. It is a daily reaffirmation that diabetic-friendly food can be incredibly delicious, profoundly nourishing, and surprisingly straightforward to prepare. So, let's reclaim lunchtime as a moment to savor, enjoy, and nurture our bodies and spirits with every bite. You won't believe how delicious these recipes are until you try them yourself!

This collection from **"Delicious Diabetic Cookbook for Beginners"** turns lunchtime into an opportunity for creativity, flavor, and nourishment. Each recipe is designed to be simple yet satisfying, perfect for anyone managing prediabetes or Type 2 diabetes. Here's to lunches that delight the senses, fuel the body, and bring joy to your day.

AVOCADO CHICKEN SALAD

Ingredients

- 2 cups shredded chicken (the tender embrace)
- 2 ripe avocados, diced (the creamy dream)
- Juice of 1 lime (a splash of zest)
- 1/4 cup cilantro, finely chopped (a hint of freshness)
- Salt and pepper, to taste (the flavor enhancers)
- Optional: diced red onion or cherry tomatoes for added color and crunch

Nutritional Information:
Per serving: Estimated values: 300 calories, 25g protein, 12g carbohydrates, 20g fat, 7g fiber, 60mg cholesterol, 200mg sodium, 700mg potassium.

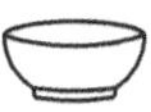  

Prep Time: 20 min

Cook Time: 0 min (assuming chicken is pre-cooked)

Serves: 4

Directions

1. **Combine with Ease:** Mix the shredded chicken and diced avocado in a large bowl. Let the creamy avocado texture and the tender chicken intertwine like old friends catching up.
2. **Dress in Zest:** Squeeze the lime juice over the mixture, ensuring every piece has kissed with its zesty cheer. It is where the salad comes alive, each bite promising a tangy delight.
3. **Sprinkle with Freshness:** Add the chopped cilantro and the diced red onion or cherry tomatoes if you're using them. Add salt and pepper, then mix everything until the salad is evenly coated with joy and flavor.
4. **Serve with Delight:** Serve the salad chilled for a refreshing lunch, or scoop it onto whole-grain bread for a heartwarming sandwich. It's perfect for a sunny day picnic or a cozy indoor brunch, bringing joy to every bite.

Summary:

This **Avocado Chicken Salad** isn't just a dish; it's a joyful reunion of flavors and textures. Each bite weaves together the tenderness of the chicken, the creamy richness of avocado, and the bright, cheerful tang of lime, all accented by the fresh, green spark of cilantro. It's a salad that celebrates simplicity and taste, that nourishes the body and delights the soul.

QUINOA VEGGIE WRAP

Ingredients

- 1 cup quinoa (the heart of the wrap)
- 2 cups water (to fluff up the quinoa)
- 1 whole-grain tortilla per serving (the cozy blanket)
- 1 cup mixed veggies (bell peppers, spinach, and cherry tomatoes, the colorful joy)
- 1/2 cup feta cheese, crumbled (the tangy surprise)
- 2 tablespoons olive oil (for sautéing veggies)
- Salt and pepper, to taste (the flavor dance)
- Optional: a drizzle of balsamic glaze or hummus for extra zing

Nutritional Information:

Per serving: Estimated values: 320 calories, 12g protein, 45g carbohydrates, 12g fat, 6g fiber, 25mg cholesterol, 400mg sodium, 300mg potassium.

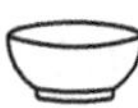  

Prep Time: 15 min   Cook Time: 20 min   Serves: 4

(for the quinoa)

Directions

1. **Quinoa's Journey:** Bring quinoa and water to a rolling boil in a saucepan, then drop the heat to a gentle simmer and cover. Cook for about 15 minutes until the quinoa puffs up. Let it sit for 5 minutes, then give it a fluffy stir with a fork.
2. **Sauté with Love:** Heat olive oil in a pan while the quinoa cooks. Add the mixed veggies, sautéing until they're tender but still vibrant. Top with crumbled feta cheese for a creamy, tangy finish.
3. **Wrap and Roll:** Lay out your whole-grain tortillas. Spoon a generous quinoa base onto each, followed by the sautéed veggies. Shower the top with crumbled feta cheese for a creamy, tangy kick.
4. **Seal the Deal:** Drizzle a bit of balsamic glaze or spread a thin layer of hummus over the veggies for extra flavor. Roll the tortillas tightly to encase the filling in a snug, delicious embrace.
5. **Serve with a Smile:** Cut each wrap in half to reveal the colorful layers of joy inside. Serve immediately or wrap them up for a nourishing meal on the go.

Summary:

The **Quinoa Veggie Wrap** is a symphony of textures and flavors, a reminder that simple ingredients can come together to create something extraordinary. Each bite is a celebration, from the fluffy quinoa that whispers comfort to the crisp veggies that sing with freshness, all tied together with the tangy notes of feta cheese.

TURMERIC LENTIL SOUP

Ingredients

- 1 cup red lentils (the heart of the soup)
- 1 large carrot, diced (a crunch of sweetness)
- 1 large onion, diced (the flavor foundation)
- 2 cloves garlic, minced (a whisper of warmth)
- 1 teaspoon of ground turmeric (the golden touch)
- 1/2 teaspoon ground cumin (a hint of the earth)
- 4 cups vegetable broth
- 1 tablespoon olive oil
- Salt and pepper, to taste
- Fresh cilantro for garnish
- **Optional:** a squeeze of lemon juice

Nutritional Information:

Per serving: Estimated values: 180 calories, 11g protein, 30g carbohydrates, 2g fat, 15g fiber, 0mg cholesterol, 300mg sodium, 600mg potassium.

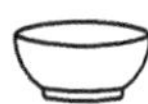  

Prep Time: 10 min   Cook Time: 30 min   Serves: 6

Directions

1. **Sauté to Start:** Heat the olive oil over medium heat in a large pot. Add the onions and carrots, sautéing until they start to soften. Stir in the garlic, turmeric, and cumin, and cook for another minute until fragrant, painting the beginnings of your soup with colors and scents.
2. **Lentils Unite:** Rinse the lentils under cold water and add them to the pot, coating them with the spiced vegetable mix. Pour the vegetable broth into the pot, letting the soup heat until it simmers.
3. **Simmer and Soften:** Allow the soup to simmer for about 25-30 minutes, or until the lentils are soft and the soup has thickened to your preference. The transformation into a comforting bowl of warmth begins.
4. **Final Flavors:** Season the soup with salt and pepper to taste. For a vibrant twist, squeeze in some lemon juice to slice through the soup's richness.
5. **Serve with Love:** Ladle the soup into bowls, garnishing each with fresh cilantro. Each spoonful is a warm embrace, a comfort in a bowl.

Summary:

Turmeric Lentil Soup is more than just a meal; it's a soothing journey, a comforting experience that warms you from the inside out. With every spoonful, the warmth of turmeric, the heartiness of lentils, and the grounding touch of carrots and onions embrace you. It's a simple yet profound soup that speaks to the soul, offering nourishment, comfort, and a golden glow of well-being. Perfect for any day, this soup is a reminder that the most comforting dishes are often the simplest.

CAPRESE ZOODLE SALAD

Ingredients

- Four medium zucchinis (the green canvas)
- 1 cup cherry tomatoes, halved (the juicy gems)
- 8 ounces fresh mozzarella, cubed or in pearls (the creamy dream)
- 1/4 cup fresh basil leaves, torn (the fragrant whisper)
- Two tablespoons of balsamic glaze (the sweet embrace)
- One tablespoon of olive oil (liquid gold)
- Salt and pepper, to taste (the flavor harmonizers)

Optional: A sprinkle of pine nuts or red pepper flakes for a bit of crunch and heat

Nutritional Information: Per serving: Estimated values: 220 calories, 14g protein, 10g carbohydrates, 15g fat, 2g fiber, 30mg cholesterol, 200mg sodium, 400mg potassium.

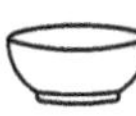  

Prep Time: 15 min   Cook Time: 0 min   Serves: 4

Directions

1. **Zoodle Creation:** Use a spiralizer to turn the zucchinis into noodles, creating a bed of green, curling zoodles that will serve as the base of your salad. It's like crafting edible green ribbons, each one a promise of freshness.
2. **Toss Together:** In a large bowl, gently toss the zoodles with cherry tomatoes, fresh mozzarella, and basil leaves. The colors and textures combine in a dance, a vibrant blend of summer's best.
3. **Dress with Love:** Drizzle the olive oil and balsamic glaze over the salad. Season the dish with salt and pepper according to your taste. Each addition is a layer of flavor, adding depth and richness to the salad's lightness.
4. **Serve with Joy:** Divide the salad among plates, ensuring each serving gets an even mix of zoodles, tomatoes, mozzarella, and basil. For a final touch, sprinkle with pine nuts or red pepper flakes.

Summary:

Caprese Zoodle Salad is a refreshing twist on a beloved classic, blending the familiar flavors of caprese with the innovative twist of zucchini noodles. Each forkful is a journey through a garden of textures and tastes, from the creamy bites of mozzarella to the burst of juicy tomatoes and the tender crispness of zoodles, all brought together with the rich sweetness of balsamic glaze. This salad is a celebration of simplicity, a dish that speaks of summer days, healthful choices, and the joy of eating food that tastes good and feels good.

CHICKPEA GREEK SALAD

Ingredients

- 2 15-ounce cans of chickpeas, rinsed and ready (the hearty stars)
- 1 large cucumber, diced (the crisp freshness)
- 1 cup cherry tomatoes, halved (the sweet bursts)
- 1/2 cup Kalamata olives, pitted (the savory whispers)
- 1/2 cup feta cheese, crumbled (the creamy dream)
- 1/4 cup red onion, thinly sliced (the flavor kick)

For the dressing:

- 1/4 cup olive oil (the golden pour)
- 2 tablespoons of red wine vinegar (the zesty tang)
- 1 teaspoon of dried oregano (the herbaceous hug)
- Salt and pepper, to taste (the perfect finish)

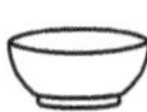  

Prep Time: 15min   Cook Time:25 min   Serves: 4

Directions

1. **Salad Symphony:** In a large bowl, combine the chickpeas, cucumber, cherry tomatoes, Kalamata olives, feta cheese, and red onion. It's like gathering friends for a celebration, each bringing a unique flavor to the party.
2. **Dress in Joy:** In a small bowl, blend red wine vinegar, dried oregano, salt, pepper, and olive oil. This dressing is the melody that brings the salad to life, each ingredient playing off the others in perfect harmony.
3. **Toss to mingle:** Pour the dressing over the salad and gently toss, making sure every chickpea, cucumber cube, and tomato slice is evenly coated with the zesty sauce.
4. **Serve with Heart:** Divide the salad among plates or bowls, serving it as a vibrant, nourishing, filling, and refreshing meal. It's a dish meant to be shared, a moment of connection over simple, wholesome food.

Nutritional Information: Per serving: Estimated values: 350 calories, 15g protein, 40g carbohydrates, 18g fat, 10g fiber, 25mg cholesterol, 700mg sodium, 400mg potassium.

Summary:

The **Chickpea Greek Salad** is more than just a dish; it celebrates flavors, textures, and colors. Each bite is a journey to the heart of Greek cuisine, reimagined through the wholesome goodness of chickpeas and the classic combination of cucumber, tomatoes, olives, and feta. The salad stands tall as a meal, offering satisfaction and joy.

TUNA AND WHITE BEAN SALAD

Ingredients

- 2 cans (every 5 ounces) of tuna in water, drained (the ocean's bounty)
- 1can (15 ounces) white beans, rinsed and drained (the creamy heart)
- 1 small red onion, finely chopped (the crisp bite)
- 1/4 cup fresh parsley, chopped (the verdant splash)
- Juice of 1 lemon (the zesty soul)
- 2 tablespoons olive oil (the golden drizzle)
- Salt and pepper, to taste (the seasoning whisper)
- Optional: Cherry tomatoes or cucumber slices

Nutritional Information:

Per serving: Estimated values: 250 calories, 22g protein, 25g carbohydrates, 7g fat, 6g fiber, 30mg cholesterol, 200mg sodium, 500mg potassium.

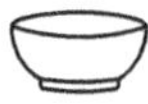  

Prep Time: 10 min   Cook Time: 0 min   Serves: 4

Directions

1. **Combine with Care:** In a large bowl, mix the tuna, white beans, red onion, and parsley. It's a gathering of simple ingredients, each bringing its own charm and flavor to the mix.
2. **Dress to Impress:** Squeeze the lemon juice over the salad, then drizzle with olive oil—season with salt and pepper. Gently toss everything together, letting the dressing coat each ingredient lovingly, bringing the salad to life.
3. **Optional Add-ins:** Now's the time to mix in cherry tomatoes or cucumber slices, tossing them in for a splash of color and crispness.
4. **Serve with Joy:** Divide the salad among plates or bowls. It's ready to eat immediately, a no-cook wonder that's as satisfying as it is simple.

Summary:

The **Tuna and White Bean Salad** celebrates simplicity and nourishment, a dish that brings together hearty beans, lean tuna, and crisp onions, all brightened by a lemony dressing. Here's to enjoying the simple pleasures of food, to lunches that energize and satisfy, and to the joy of eating well every day.

TURKEY AND APPLE SANDWICH

Ingredients

- 4 slices of whole-grain bread (the sturdy, heart-healthy foundation)
- 4 ounces thinly sliced turkey breast (the lean, savory star)
- 1 medium apple, cored and thinly sliced (the crisp, sweet contrast)
- 2 tablespoons mustard (the bold, zesty companion)
- Lettuce leaves (the fresh, crunchy layer)
- Optional: a sprinkle of black pepper or thin slices of red onion for an extra flavor kick

Nutritional Information:

Per serving: Estimated values: 350 calories, 25g protein, 45g carbohydrates, 5g fat, 6g fiber, 30mg cholesterol, 680mg sodium, 300mg potassium.

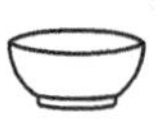  

Prep Time: 5 min   Cook Time: 0 min   Serves: 2

Directions

1. **Lay the Foundation:** Start with laying out your slices of whole-grain bread. Whole-grain bread isn't just bread; it's a canvas waiting for its masterpiece. And this masterpiece is easy to create, even for novice cooks.
2. **Spread the Joy:** On two slices of bread, spread the mustard evenly. The mustard isn't just a condiment here; it's the zesty heart of this culinary creation, ready to tie all the flavors together.
3. **Layer the Love:** On top of the mustard-spread slices, arrange the thinly sliced turkey, followed by apple slices. The turkey brings a gentle, savory flavor that perfectly complements the sweet, crisp notes of the apple.
4. **Final Touches:** Add lettuce leaves for a fresh crunch. If you're feeling adventurous, a sprinkle of black pepper or a few slices of red onion can add an extra dimension of flavor.
5. **Close and Enjoy:** Top with the remaining slices of bread. Press gently, slice the sandwich in half, and behold the beauty of simple, wholesome ingredients coming together.

Summary:

The **Turkey and Apple Sandwich** is more than just a meal; it's a delightful journey through textures and tastes. Each bite is a celebration of balance, a sweet and savory embrace that satisfies every taste bud.

Roasted Veggie Hummus Wrap

Ingredients

- 4 spinach tortillas (the vibrant embrace)
- 1 cup hummus (the creamy heart)
- 1 red bell pepper, sliced (the sweet crunch)
- 1 zucchini, sliced (the summer whisper)
- 1 yellow squash, sliced (the golden touch)
- 1 small red onion, sliced (the flavor spark)
- 2 tablespoons olive oil (the golden drizzle)
- Salt and pepper, to taste
- **Optional:** feta cheese, sun-dried tomatoes, or arugula for an extra layer of flavor

Nutritional Information:
Per serving: Estimated values: 320 calories, 10g protein, 45g carbohydrates, 12g fat, 8g fiber, 0mg cholesterol, 580mg sodium, 400mg potassium.

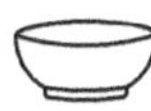  

Prep Time: 15min   Cook Time:25 min   Serves: 4

Directions

1. **Roast to Perfection:** Preheat your oven to 400°F (200°C). Slather a thick layer of hummus on each tortilla, creating the perfect base for your roasted veggies. Spread them out and roast until they're tender and sweetly browned, about 25 minutes, turning them into roasted delights.
2. **Warm and Spread:** Warm the spinach tortillas slightly to make them more pliable. Spread a rich layer of hummus on each tortilla, setting the stage for your roasted veggies.
3. **Layer and Love:** Once the vegetables have roasted to perfection, spread them evenly across the hummus-slathered tortillas. Sprinkle feta cheese, sun-dried tomatoes, or a handful of arugulas over the veggies for added flavor and texture.
4. **Wrap and Serve:** Tightly roll up the tortillas, tucking in the sides as you go, to snugly encase the filling in a delicious embrace. Cut each wrap in half diagonally, revealing the colorful cross-section of veggies and hummus.

Summary:

The **Roasted Veggie Hummus Wrap** is a love letter to the simple joy of eating. It combines the earthy goodness of roasted seasonal vegetables with the creamy richness of hummus, all rolled up in a spinach tortilla that adds a touch of joy with every bite. This wrap is a testament to the beauty of wholesome ingredients coming together in harmony, offering a meal that's not only delicious but also nourishing. It's perfect for a quick lunch, a picnic treat, or anytime you need a little reminder of how delightful eating well can be.

Shrimp and Avocado Salad

Ingredients

- 1 pound cooked shrimp, peeled and deveined (the ocean's bounty)
- 2 ripe avocados, diced (the creamy delight)
- 1 mango, diced (the tropical sweetness)
- 1/4 cup red onion, finely chopped (the sharp contrast)
- 1/4 cup cilantro, chopped (the fresh burst)
- Juice of 2 limes (the zesty dressing)
- 2 tablespoons olive oil (the smooth binder)
- Salt and pepper, to taste (the flavor enhancers)
- **Optional:** chili flakes

Nutritional Information:
Per serving: Estimated values: 320 calories, 24g protein, 20g carbohydrates, 18g fat, 7g fiber, 180mg cholesterol, 300mg sodium, 800mg potassium.

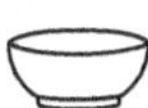  

Prep Time: 15 min   Cook Time: 5 min   Serves: 4

Directions

1. **Prepare the Ingredients:** If your shrimp remains undercooked, boil or grill it until pink and set aside to cool. Meanwhile, dice the avocados and mango into bite-sized pieces.
2. **Mix the Dressing:** In a small bowl, whisk together lime juice, olive oil, salt, and pepper. This simple citrus dressing will tie all the flavors together beautifully.
3. **Combine the Salad:** In a large mixing bowl, combine the cooked shrimp, diced avocados, mango, red onion, and cilantro. Drizzle the dressing over the top and gently toss to coat all the ingredients without breaking the avocado.
4. **Serve Fresh:** To keep the ingredients fresh and vibrant, serve the salad immediately after preparing it. Add a sprinkle of chili flakes if you like a bit of heat.
5. **Enjoy:** Dig into this refreshing salad bursting with flavors and textures. It's perfect for a healthy lunch or a side dish at dinner.

Summary:

This **Shrimp and Avocado Salad** is not just a meal; it's a vibrant celebration of fresh, wholesome ingredients. Juicy shrimp paired with creamy avocado and sweet mango offers a delightful contrast of flavors and textures, all brought together with a tangy lime dressing. It's a perfect dish for anyone looking for a nutritious, delicious, quick-to-prepare meal that's as suitable for a busy weekday as it is for a leisurely weekend lunch. Here's to the joy of eating food that's as good for the body as it is pleasing to the palate.

Soba Noodle Salad with Peanut Dressing

Ingredients

- 8 oz soba noodles (the earthy foundation)
- 1 cup shredded carrots (the sweet crunch)
- 1 cup sliced cucumber (the fresh splash)
- 1 red bell pepper, thinly sliced (the vibrant cheer)
- 1/4 cup chopped green onions (the sharp spark)
- 1/4 cup chopped cilantro (the fragrant kiss)

For the Peanut Dressing:

- 1/4 cup peanut butter (the creamy heart)
- 2 tablespoons soy sauce (the umami depth)
- 1 tablespoon of rice vinegar (the zesty lift)
- 1 tablespoon of honey (the subtle sweetness)
- 1 teaspoon of sesame oil (the nutty whisper)
- 1 teaspoon of grated ginger (the spicy warmth)
- Water to thin, as needed

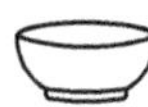  

Prep Time: 20 min   Cook Time: 8 min   Serves: 4

Directions

1. **Noodle Dance:** Cook soba noodles according to package instructions, aiming for al dente. Rinse under cold water to chill and stop cooking, then drain well. It's the beginning of a beautiful salad story.
2. **Veggie Rainbow:** In a large bowl, combine the chilled noodles with shredded carrots, sliced cucumber, red bell pepper, green onions, and cilantro. Each ingredient adds color and texture to the salad, like brush strokes on a canvas.
3. **Dressing Dream:** Whisk peanut butter, soy sauce, rice vinegar, honey, sesame oil, and grated ginger until smooth. Suppose the dressing is too thick. Thin it with water to achieve your desired consistency. This dressing is the melody that brings the salad to life, rich and embracing.
4. **Toss to Perfection:** Pour the peanut dressing over the noodle and vegetable mixture, tossing gently to coat everything. This moment is one of harmony, where every element of the salad comes together.
5. **Serve with Love:** Divide the salad among plates or bowls, garnishing with additional cilantro or green onions if desired. Each bite is a journey through flavors and textures, a delightful experience of the senses.

Nutritional Information: Per serving: Estimated values: 320 calories, 10g protein, 50g carbohydrates, 12g fat, 6g fiber, 0mg cholesterol, 620mg sodium, 400mg potassium.

Summary:

Soba Noodle Salad with Peanut Dressing is a delightful mix of tastes and textures, featuring rich, earthy noodles alongside crisp, fresh veggies, all bound together with a luscious, spicy peanut sauce. It's a salad that tells a story of balance and harmony, inviting you on a culinary journey that's both nourishing and delightfully satisfying. Here's to meals that celebrate the diversity of ingredients, the joy of mixing traditions and flavors, and the simple pleasure of a dish that's as beautiful to look at as it is to eat.

BUTTERNUT SQUASH SOUP

Ingredients

- 1 medium butternut squash, peeled, seeded, and cubed (the golden heart)
- 1 tablespoon of olive oil (the smooth glaze)
- 1 medium onion, chopped (the flavor foundation)
- 2 cloves garlic, minced (the aroma lifts)
- 1 teaspoon of grated ginger (the spicy whisper)
- A pinch of nutmeg (the warm embrace)
- 4 cups vegetable broth (the soothing liquid)
- Salt and pepper, to taste (the seasoning soul)
- Optional: a swirl of cream or a sprinkle of pumpkin seeds for garnish (the finishing touch)

Nutritional Information: Per serving: Estimated values: 180 calories, 3g protein, 30g carbohydrates, 5g fat, 6g fiber, 0mg cholesterol, 500mg sodium, 500mg potassium.

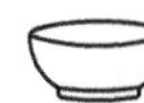  

Prep Time: 15 min   Cook Time: 45 min   Serves: 4

Directions

1. **Roast to Perfection:** Toss the butternut squash cubes with olive oil and spread them on a baking sheet—roast at 400°F for 25 minutes or until tender and caramelized, unlocking their natural sweetness and depth.
2. **Sauté the Base:** In a large pot, sauté the onion until translucent. Add the garlic and ginger, cooking for another minute until fragrant. It's the start of something comforting, base rich with flavors.
3. **Blend the Warmth:** Add the roasted butternut squash to the pot and the vegetable broth, nutmeg, salt, and pepper. Bring to a simmer, then blend until smooth, using an immersion blender or carefully transferring to a blender in batches.
4. **Simmer to Merge:** Let the soup simmer for another 10 minutes, allowing the flavors to marry and the soup to reach the perfect creamy consistency. It's a gentle process, a harmonious blend of ingredients.
5. **Serve with Love:** Ladle the soup into bowls, garnishing with a swirl of cream or a sprinkle of pumpkin seeds if desired. Each bowl is a warm hug, a comforting blend of sweetness and spice.

Summary:

Butternut Squash Soup is more than just a meal; it's comfort in liquid form, a bowl of warmth that wraps its arms around you with every spoonful. From the roasting of the squash that fills your kitchen with the scent of autumn to the final swirl of cream that adds just the right touch of decadence, it's a culinary journey that's as satisfying to create as it is to consume. This soup is a reminder of the simple pleasures in life, the joy in the flavors of the season, and the warmth that comes from sharing a meal made with love. Here's to the soups that soothe our souls and warm our hearts.

MEDITERRANEAN CHICKPEA SALAD

Ingredients

- 2 cans (15 ounces each) of chickpeas, drained and rinsed (the stars of the show)
- 1 cucumber diced (the cool crunch)
- 1/2 cup pitted and sliced Kalamata olives (the salty jewels)
- 1 cup cherry tomatoes, halved (the sweet bursts)
- 1/4 cup red onion, thinly sliced (the sharp contrast)
- 1/4 cup of extra virgin olive oil (the liquid gold)
- Juice of 1 lemon (the zesty soul)
- 1 teaspoon of dried oregano (the aromatic whisper)
- Salt and pepper, to taste (the flavor enhancers)
- Fresh parsley, chopped, for garnish (the green flourish)

Nutritional Information:
Per serving: Estimated values: 250 calories, 10g protein, 35g carbohydrates, 10g fat, 9g fiber, 0mg cholesterol, 300mg sodium, 400mg potassium.

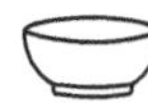  

Prep Time: 15 min   Cook Time: 0 min   Serves: 4

Directions

1. **Toss Together:** In a large mixing bowl, combine the chickpeas, cucumber, cherry tomatoes, Kalamata olives, and red onion. It's like gathering friends for a colorful, joyful feast under the Mediterranean sun.
2. **Make the Dressing:** Combine dried oregano, salt, and pepper in a small bowl, mix with olive oil and lemon juice, and whisk until the ingredients are fully blended into a smooth dressing. This dressing is the magic that will tie all the salad ingredients together, each drop infused with the flavors of the Mediterranean.
3. **Dress and Mix:** Pour the dressing over the salad ingredients, gently tossing to ensure every chickpea and cucumber slice is coated in the lemony, herby dressing. Lovingly coat each tomato half in the dressing.
4. **Garnish and Serve:** Sprinkle the chopped fresh parsley over the salad, adding a pop of color and a fresh, vibrant flavor that complements the salad perfectly.
5. **Enjoy:** Chill the salad at room temperature to best appreciate the mix of flavors and textures. It's not just a salad; it's a Mediterranean adventure in a bowl.

Summary:

The **Mediterranean Chickpea Salad** is more than just a dish; it's a celebration of vibrant flavors and nourishing ingredients, a testament to the simplicity and richness of Mediterranean cuisine. Every bite is a delightful experience, blending textures and tastes that transport you to sunny shores and lush gardens. It's a salad that nourishes both body and soul, reminding us of the joys of eating food that is not only good for us but also incredibly delicious. Here's to meals that bring us a little closer to the beauty and abundance of the Mediterranean.

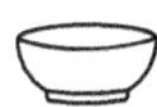  

Ingredients

- 4 boneless, skinless chicken breasts (the canvas)
- 2 cups fresh spinach, chopped (the vibrant green)
- 1/2 cup feta cheese, crumbled (the creamy dream)
- 2 cloves garlic, minced (the flavor spark)
- 1 tablespoon of olive oil (for cooking and flavor)
- Salt and pepper, to taste (the seasoning duo)
- Toothpicks (to secure the masterpiece)

Nutritional Information:

Per serving: Estimated values: 290 calories, 35g protein, 5g carbohydrates, 15g fat, 2g fiber, 75mg cholesterol, 590mg sodium, 450mg potassium

Prep Time: 20 min   Cook Time: 25 min   Serves: 4

Directions

1. **Get started:** Prepare oven: heat to 375°F (190°C). While the oven warms, gently pound the chicken breasts to an even thickness to make them more pliable for stuffing.
2. **Sauté to Soften:** Heat a skillet with a tablespoon of olive oil over medium heat. Sauté the garlic briefly until fragrant, then add the spinach and cook until just wilted. It's a quick dance in the pan, a whirlwind of greens turning tender and aromatic.
3. **Stuff and Secure:** Lay the chicken breasts flat and season each with salt and pepper. Heap a good spoonful of the spinach mixture onto each chicken breast and top with feta cheese. Roll up the chicken around the filling and use toothpicks to secure the rolls.
4. **Bake to Perfection:** Place the stuffed chicken breasts seam-side down in a baking dish. Bake in the warmed oven for about 25 minutes or until the chicken is cooked and the juices clear. It's a waiting game, anticipation building with the aroma filling the kitchen.
5. **Serve with Love:** Remove the toothpicks, then slice the chicken rolls to reveal the creamy, colorful filling. Serve hot, each slice a testament to the joy of cooking and the beauty of simple, flavorful ingredients coming together in perfect harmony.

Summary:

The **Spinach and Feta Stuffed Chicken Breast** is a dish that sings with flavors, a symphony of juicy chicken, creamy feta, and tender spinach, all wrapped up in a tender embrace. It's a meal that feels like a celebration, a burst of taste and texture that's both comforting and exhilarating. Each bite is a journey, a discovery of layers and depth that delights and satisfies. Here's to meals that bring us together, to flavors that tell a story, and to the simple joy of a dish made with love and care.

COLD ASIAN NOODLE SALAD

Ingredients

- 8 oz whole wheat spaghetti (the hearty base)
- 1 large carrot, julienned (the vibrant crunch)
- 1 red bell pepper julienned (the sweet pop)
- 1 yellow bell pepper, julienned (the sunny addition)
- 1/4 cup chopped fresh cilantro (the fresh twist)

For the Sesame-Ginger Dressing:

- 3 tablespoons sesame oil (the smooth richness)
- 2 tablespoons soy sauce (the umami depth)
- 1 tablespoon of rice vinegar (the tangy lift)
- 2 teaspoons of freshly grated ginger (the zesty spice)
- 1 garlic clove, minced (the flavor burst)
- 1 tablespoon of honey (a touch of sweetness)
- Optional: Add a dash of sesame seeds or crushed peanuts for a decorative touch.

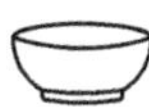  

Prep Time: 15 min   Cook Time: 10 min   Serves: 4

Directions

1. **Cook Spaghetti:** Boil the whole wheat spaghetti according to the package instructions until al dente. Drain and rinse under cold water to cool. Set aside to drain thoroughly.
2. **Prepare Vegetables:** While the spaghetti cooks, julienne the carrots and bell peppers, ensuring each strip is thin and uniform to embrace each dressing note perfectly.
3. **Whisk Dressing:** In a small bowl, combine sesame oil, soy sauce, rice vinegar, grated ginger, minced garlic, and honey. Whisk the ingredients until they blend into a harmonious dressing.
4. **Combine Ingredients:** In a large mixing bowl, toss the cooled spaghetti with the julienned vegetables and chopped cilantro. Gently pour the dressing over the salad and lightly toss until evenly coated.
5. **Serve Chilled:** Refrigerate the salad for at least 30 minutes before serving to intensify the flavors and blend perfectly. Garnish with sesame seeds or crushed peanuts just before serving for added texture and flair.

Nutritional Information:

Per serving: Estimated values: 320 calories, 10g protein, 55g carbohydrates, 9g fat, 8g fiber, 0mg cholesterol, 320mg sodium, 350mg potassium.

Summary:

This **Cold Asian Noodle Salad** is a mix of various textures and tastes, creating the ideal dish for a refreshing lunch or a breezy summer evening meal. Whole wheat spaghetti provides a fiber-rich base, while the crisp vegetables add color and crunch. The sesame-ginger dressing infuses each bite with depth and zest. This salad celebrates fresh ingredients and vibrant tastes, ideal for a nutritious yet satisfying meal.

Lentil and Sweet Potato Chili

Ingredients

- 1 tablespoon olive oil (the silky start)
- 1 large onion, chopped (the flavor foundation)
- 2 cloves garlic, minced (the aromatic enhancers)
- 2 large, sweet potatoes, peeled and cubed (the hearty soul)
- 1 cup dried lentils, rinsed (the robust heart)
- 1 red bell pepper, diced (the sweet crunch)
- 2 tablespoons chili powder (the spicy kick)
- 1 teaspoon of cumin (the smoky whisper)
- 1/2 teaspoon paprika (the subtle warmth)
- 4 cups vegetable broth (the comforting base)
- 1 can (28 ounces) of crushed tomatoes (the rich backdrop)
- Salt and pepper, to taste (the essential seasoners)
- Fresh cilantro, chopped, for garnish (the fresh finish)

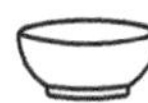  

Prep Time: 15 min   Cook Time: 40 min   Serves: 6

Directions

1. **Sauté the Base:** Heat the olive oil over medium heat in a large pot. Add the chopped onion and garlic, sautéing until they are translucent and fragrant, setting the stage for a dish full of depth and flavor.
2. **Simmer the Heart:** Add the sweet potatoes, lentils, and red bell pepper to the pot, stirring to combine. Sprinkle in the chili powder, cumin, and paprika, evenly coating the vegetables and lentils. Cook for a few minutes until the spices are fragrant.
3. **Pour and Boil:** Add the vegetable broth and crushed tomatoes to the pot. Heat the mixture until it bubbles, then reduce the heat and let it softly simmer for about 30 minutes, making sure the lentils and sweet potatoes soften.
4. **Season and Serve:** Season the chili with salt and pepper to taste. Let the chili stand for a few minutes off the heat to thicken slightly, enhancing its rich, hearty texture.
5. **Garnish and Enjoy:** Ladle the chili into bowls and garnish with chopped fresh cilantro. Each spoonful is a burst of flavors, from the earthiness of the lentils to the sweetness of the sweet potatoes, all wrapped in a tangy tomato embrace.

Nutritional Information:

Per serving: Estimated values: 290 calories, 12g protein, 54g carbohydrates, 4g fat, 15g fiber, 0mg cholesterol, 700mg sodium, 800mg potassium.

Summary:

Lentil and Sweet Potato Chili is not just a meal; it's a comforting embrace on a chilly day, a bowl of rich, robust flavors that are nourishing and satisfying. This chili is a testament to the power of combining simple ingredients to create something wonderfully complex and delightful. It's perfect for warming up after a long day, serving at gatherings, or enjoying a cozy meal that feeds the body and the spirit. Here's to the joys of hearty chili, its comfort, and the smiles it gathers around the table.

CAULIFLOWER RICE STIR-FRY

Ingredients

- 1 large head of cauliflower, grated into rice-like granules (the versatile star)
- 2 tablespoons sesame oil (for sautéing and flavor)
- 1 cup mixed bell peppers, thinly sliced (the color pops)
- 1/2 cup carrots, julienned (the sweet crunch)
- 1/2 cup snap peas (the crisp addition)
- 2 green onions, sliced (the sharp bite)
- 2 cloves garlic, minced (the flavor booster)
- 1 tablespoon of fresh ginger, minced (the zesty spark)
- 2 tablespoons soy sauce (the umami depth)
- 1 tablespoon of oyster sauce (optional for richness)
- Salt and pepper, to taste (the seasoning duo)
- Optional: a sprinkle of sesame seeds or chopped cilantro for garnish

Nutritional Information:

Per serving: Estimated values: 150 calories, 4g protein, 18g carbohydrates, 7g fat, 5g fiber, 0mg cholesterol, 600mg sodium, 300mg potassium.

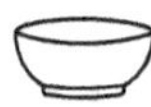  

Prep Time: 10 min   Cook Time: 15 min   Serves: 4

Directions

1. **Prepare Cauliflower Rice:** Wash and dry the cauliflower head. Cut the ingredients into chunks, pulse them in a food processor, and wait until they resemble rice grains. This base will carry all the wonderful flavors of your stir-fry.
2. **Heat and Sauté:** Heat the sesame oil in a sizable skillet or wok on medium-high heat until it glistens. Add the minced garlic and ginger, sautéing briefly until aromatic—this is where the magic begins.
3. **Veggie Medley:** Add the bell peppers, carrots, and snap peas to the skillet. Stir-fry for about 5 minutes until they're just tender but still have a bite. This step builds the foundation of your dish with vibrant veggies.
4. **Add Cauliflower Rice:** Blend the cauliflower rice into the skillet, ensuring you distribute it evenly among the vegetables. Cook for about 5-7 minutes, allowing the cauliflower to soften slightly and brown, picking up all the beautiful flavors in the pan.
5. **Season Perfectly:** Pour the soy sauce and oyster sauce (if using) into the skillet, then season with salt and pepper to taste. Stir everything to combine and coat evenly. Cook for about an additional 2 minutes to let the flavors meld together.
6. **Garnish and Serve:** Remove from heat. Serve your Cauliflower Rice Stir-Fry garnished with sesame seeds or chopped cilantro for extra flavor and freshness.

Summary:

This **Cauliflower Rice Stir-Fry** is not just a meal; it's a celebration of textures and flavors, bringing together the lightness of cauliflower with the hearty crunch of fresh vegetables, all tied together with rich, savory sauces. It's a perfect example of how low-carb can still mean high flavor, making it an ideal choice for anyone looking to satisfy their stir-fry cravings without guilt. Here's to enjoying a dish that's as nourishing as it is delicious, proving that healthy eating doesn't have to be boring.

STUFFED BELL PEPPERS

Ingredients

- 4 large bell peppers, tops cut off and seeds removed (the colorful vessels)
- 1 tablespoon olive oil (the healthy sauté base)
- 1 onion, finely chopped (the flavor foundation)
- 2 cloves garlic, minced (the aromatic touch)
- 1/2 pound ground turkey (the lean protein)
- 1 cup cooked quinoa (the nutritious filler)
- 1 can (14.5 ounces) diced tomatoes, drained (the juicy component)
- 1 teaspoon dried oregano (the herby hint)
- 1 teaspoon of dried basil (the fragrant boost)
- Salt and pepper, to taste (the essential seasonings)
- 1/2 cup shredded mozzarella cheese (optional for topping)

Nutritional Information:

Per serving: Estimated values: 290 calories, 18g protein, 30g carbohydrates, 10g fat, 6g fiber, 45mg cholesterol, 400mg sodium, 700mg potassium.

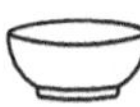  

Prep Time: 20 min   Cook Time: 40 min   Serves: 4

Directions

1. **Preheat Oven and Prepare Peppers:** Preheat your oven to 375°F (190°C). Prepare the bell peppers by removing the tops and scooping out the seeds. Set aside the cleaned peppers.
2. **Cook the Filling:** Heat olive oil over medium heat in a skillet. Add the chopped onion and minced garlic, cooking until the onion is translucent. Add the ground turkey and cook until browned, breaking it up as it cooks.
3. **Combine Ingredients:** Stir in the cooked quinoa, diced tomatoes, oregano, and basil into the turkey mixture—season with salt and pepper to taste. Cook the mixture for a few more minutes until everything is well combined and heated.
4. **Stuff the Peppers:** Spoon the mixture into each prepared bell pepper, packing it tightly. Place the stuffed peppers standing up in a baking dish.
5. **Bake:** If using, sprinkle the tops of the stuffed peppers with mozzarella cheese. Bake in the oven for about 30 minutes or until the peppers are tender and the cheese is bubbly and golden.
6. **Serve:** Let the peppers cool slightly before serving to allow the flavors to meld together. Enjoy the warmth and richness of each bite!

Summary:

Stuffed Bell Peppers are a delightful treat, each pepper a bright and cheerful vessel brimming with a savory, hearty filling. The combination of lean ground turkey and quinoa offers a high-protein, nutritious meal, while the herbs and tomatoes add layers of flavor that satisfy each bite. This dish nourishes the body and comforts the soul with its warm, home-cooked essence and vibrant presentation. It's perfect for a family dinner, offering a delicious way to enjoy a balanced, satisfying, and health-conscious meal. Here's to enjoying the simple pleasures of a well-stuffed pepper!

Kale and White Bean Soup

Ingredients

- 1 tablespoon olive oil (the smooth start)
- 1 large onion, chopped (the flavor base)
- 2 garlic cloves, minced (the aromatic touch)
- 3 large carrots, diced (the sweet crunch)
- 4 cups chopped kale (the nutrient-packed star)
- 1 can (15 ounces) white beans, drained and rinsed (the hearty element)
- 6 cups vegetable broth
- 1 teaspoon of dried thyme
- Salt and pepper, to taste
- **Optional:** Parmesan cheese for garnish

Nutritional Information:

Per serving: Estimated values: 180 calories, 10g protein, 27g carbohydrates, 4g fat, 8g fiber, 0mg cholesterol, 300mg sodium, 600mg potassium.

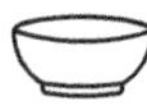  

Prep Time: 10 min   Cook Time: 30 min   Serves: 6

Directions

1. **Sauté Base Ingredients:** Heat the olive oil over medium heat in a large pot. Add the chopped onion and minced garlic, and sauté until the onion becomes translucent and the garlic is fragrant for about 5 minutes.
2. **Add Vegetables:** Stir in the diced carrots and cook for another 5 minutes until they soften. It builds a sweet and tender foundation for the soup.
3. **Simmer the Soup:** Add the chopped kale, white beans, and vegetable broth to the pot—season with dried thyme, salt, and pepper. Bring the mixture to a boil, then reduce the heat and let it simmer for about 20 minutes, or until the vegetables are tender and the flavors have melded together beautifully.
4. **Final Touches:** Adjust the seasoning if necessary. The soup should be a harmonious blend of earthy, savory, and slightly herbal flavors.
5. **Serve with Love:** Ladle the soup into bowls, and if desired, garnish with grated Parmesan cheese for a salty, umami-packed finish. Serve hot.

Summary:

Kale and White Bean Soup is a bowl of comfort, combining robust kale and creamy white beans with the sweetness of carrots, all simmered in a savory broth seasoned to perfection. This soup is more than just a meal; it's a hug in a bowl, offering warmth and nourishment with every spoonful. It's perfect for chilly evenings, leisurely lunches, or any time you need a satisfying dish packed with nutrients and flavor. Here's to the soups that make us feel at home no matter where we are.

Creamy Pumpkin Soup

Ingredients

- 2 tablespoons olive oil (the smooth beginning)
- 1 onion, finely chopped (the subtle base)
- 2 cloves garlic, minced (the flavor enhancer)
- 4 cups pumpkin puree (fresh or canned for ease)
- 4 cups vegetable broth (the gentle simmer)
- 1 teaspoon of dried sage (the earthy touch)
- 1/4 teaspoon ground nutmeg (the warm spice)
- 1 cup light cream or coconut milk (for creaminess)
- Salt and pepper, to taste
- Fresh sage leaves for garnish

Nutritional Information:

Per serving: Estimated values: 250 calories, 3g protein, 30g carbohydrates, 14g fat, 6g fiber, 20mg cholesterol, 480mg sodium, 350mg potassium.

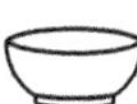  

Prep Time: 10 min   Cook Time: 30 min   Serves: 4

Directions

1. **Sauté Base:** Heat the olive oil in a large pot over medium heat. Add the chopped onion and minced garlic, cooking until the onion becomes translucent and soft, about 5 minutes.
2. **Simmer Pumpkin:** Stir in the pumpkin puree and vegetable broth—season with dried sage, nutmeg, salt, and pepper. Bring to a boil, then reduce the heat and let it simmer for about 20 minutes, allowing the flavors to meld together.
3. **Blend for Creaminess:** Blend the soup directly in the pot using an immersion blender until smooth. Do this step in batches using a regular blender for a lighter texture.
4. **Add Creaminess:** Stir in the cream or coconut milk and heat through for about 5 minutes, being careful not to boil.
5. **Serve Warm:** Ladle the soup into bowls, garnish with fresh sage leaves, and serve warm.

Summary:

This **Creamy Pumpkin Soup** is a bowl of pure comfort. It features the rich, sweet flavors of pumpkin paired with aromatic sage and warming nutmeg. It's the perfect dish to warm up a chilly day, offering a smooth, velvety texture that feels like a cozy hug. Adding cream or coconut milk adds the right touch of luxurious creaminess, making this soup a nutritious choice and a delightfully indulgent experience. Here's to enjoying fall flavors in the most comforting way possible.

ZUCCHINI BOAT PIZZAS

Ingredients

- 4 medium zucchini (the fresh vessels)
- 1 cup pizza sauce (the flavorful base)
- 1 cup shredded mozzarella cheese (the melty delight)
- 1/2 cup mini pepperoni slices or other toppings of your choice (the customizable fun)
- 1/4 cup chopped bell peppers (for a crunch)
- 1/4 cup sliced black olives (the briny contrast)
- One teaspoon of Italian seasoning
- Salt and pepper, to taste
- Fresh basil leaves for garnish

Nutritional Information:

Per serving: Estimated values: 220 calories, 12g protein, 15g carbohydrates, 14g fat, 4g fiber, 30mg cholesterol, 580mg sodium, 500mg potassium.

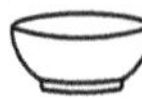  

Prep Time: 10 min   Cook Time: 20 min   Serves: 4

Directions

1. **Prepare the Zucchini:** Preheat your oven to 400°F (200°C). Slice the zucchini in half lengthwise, using a spoon to scoop out the seeds, creating a shallow cavity in each half. Lightly season with salt and pepper.
2. **Fill Them Up:** Spread pizza sauce evenly within each zucchini half. Sprinkle with mozzarella cheese, then add toppings like pepperoni, bell peppers, and olives. Sprinkle Italian seasoning over the top for an extra flavor boost.
3. **Bake to Perfection:** Arrange the zucchini boats on a baking sheet and bake in the oven for about 20 minutes until the zucchini is tender and the cheese is bubbly and golden.
4. **Garnish and Serve:** Remove from the oven and let cool for a few minutes. Garnish with fresh basil leaves for a vibrant, fresh touch. Serve hot, diving into the cheesy, saucy goodness.

Summary:

Zucchini Boat Pizzas turn a simple zucchini into a festive, fun, and flavorful meal that's both nourishing and satisfying. These boats are a playful twist on traditional pizza, offering a low-carb option that doesn't skimp on taste. The combination of melty cheese, savory toppings, and fresh, crisp zucchini is a joy.

VEGAN TACO SALAD

Ingredients

- 1 cup walnuts (the hearty base)
- 1 tablespoon soy sauce (for umami depth)
- 1 teaspoon of chili powder (the spicy kick)
- 1/2 teaspoon cumin (the smoky note)
- 1 ripe avocado, diced (the creamy delight)
- 1 cup cherry tomatoes, halved (the juicy bursts)
- 4 cups mixed greens (the leafy canvas)
- 1/4 cup red onion, finely chopped (the sharp accent)

For the Lime Vinaigrette:

- Juice of 2 limes (the tangy star)
- 3 tablespoons olive oil
- 1 teaspoon agave syrup
- Salt and pepper, to taste

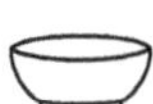  

Prep Time: 15 min   Cook Time: 0 min   Serves: 4

Directions

1. **Prepare Walnut "Meat":** In a food processor, process the walnuts until they achieve a coarse texture. Transfer to a bowl and stir in soy sauce, chili powder, and cumin. Mix until the walnuts are evenly coated with the seasonings, mimicking the texture of ground meat.
2. **Whisk the Dressing:** In a small bowl, combine lime juice, olive oil, agave syrup, salt, and pepper. Whisk until thoroughly emulsified. This zesty vinaigrette will add a vibrant, fresh flavor to the salad.
3. **Assemble the Salad:** In a large salad bowl, toss the mixed greens with red onion, cherry tomatoes, and diced avocado. Add the seasoned walnut mixture and toss lightly to combine without crushing the avocado.
4. **Dress and Serve:** Drizzle the lime vinaigrette over the salad just before serving and give it one final toss to coat everything beautifully.
5. **Enjoy Fresh:** Serve immediately, enjoying the textures and flavors that make this salad a delightful, satisfying meal.

Nutritional Information:

Per serving: Estimated values: 330 calories, 8g protein, 18g carbohydrates, 27g fat, 6g fiber, 0mg cholesterol, 200mg sodium, 600mg potassium.

Summary:

This **Vegan Taco Salad** redefines taco night with a creative twist that's visually appealing and packed with flavors and nutrients. The walnut "meat" brings a satisfying texture and spicy taste that pairs perfectly with the creamy avocado and the tangy lime vinaigrette, making every bite a delightful experience.

RATATOUILLE WITH GRILLED CHICKEN

Ingredients

- 1 chicken breast, boneless and skinless (the lean protein)
- 2 tablespoons olive oil (divided for grilling and cooking)
- 1 small eggplant, cubed (the hearty texture)
- 1 zucchini, sliced (the summer touch)
- 1 yellow squash sliced (the bright note)
- 1 red bell pepper, sliced (the sweet pop)
- 1 onion, sliced (the flavor base)
- 3 cloves garlic, minced (the aromatic kick)
- 1 can (14 ounces) of crushed tomatoes (the saucy binder)
- 1 teaspoon of dried thyme (the herby whisper)
- 1 teaspoon of dried basil (the fragrant boost)
- Salt and pepper, to taste (the seasoning duo)
- Fresh basil, chopped (for garnish)

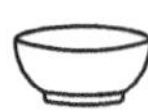

Prep Time: 20 min   Cook Time: 45 min   Serves: 4

Directions

1. **Prep Chicken:** Season chicken breasts with salt and pepper. Heat one tablespoon of olive oil in a grill pan over medium-high heat. Grill the chicken breasts until golden and cooked, about 6-7 minutes per side. Set aside and keep warm.
2. **Cook Ratatouille:** Heat the olive oil over medium heat in a large skillet. Add the onion and garlic, sautéing until the onion is translucent. Add eggplant, zucchini, yellow squash, and red bell pepper. Cook, stirring occasionally, until the vegetables are tender, about 10 minutes.
3. **Simmer with Tomatoes and Herbs:** Stir in the crushed tomatoes, thyme, and basil—season with salt and pepper. Reduce heat to low and let the ratatouille simmer for about 15 minutes, allowing the flavors to meld together.
4. **Combine and Serve:** Slice the grilled chicken breasts and arrange them on plates. Spoon the ratatouille alongside the chicken. Garnish with fresh basil before serving.
5. **Enjoy:** This wholesome meal brings a taste of France to your table, combining the rustic charm of ratatouille with the simple elegance of grilled chicken.

Nutritional Information:

Per serving: Estimated values: 320 calories, 35g protein, 20g carbohydrates, 12g fat, 6g fiber, 85mg cholesterol, 300mg sodium, 800mg potassium.

Summary:

Ratatouille with Grilled Chicken is a dish that marries rustic comfort with wholesome nutrition. The vibrant ratatouille, full of tender vegetables stewed together with herbs and tomatoes, perfectly complements the grilled chicken, offering a protein-rich meal that is both satisfying and heart-healthy. This dish nourishes the body and pleases the palate with its layers of texture and flavor. Here's to a meal celebrating good health, great taste, and the joy of eating well.

BALSAMIC BEET AND GOAT CHEESE SALAD RECIPE

Ingredients

- 4 medium beets peeled and cut into cubes (the earthy base)
- 1 tablespoon of olive oil (for roasting)
- Salt and pepper for seasoning (the flavor builders)
- 4 cups of mixed salad greens (the leafy backdrop)
- 1/2 cup goat cheese, crumbled (the creamy highlight)
- 1/4 cup toasted, sliced walnuts (the nutty accent)
- **For the Balsamic Dressing:**
- Three tablespoons of balsamic vinegar (the bold centerpiece)
- One tablespoon of Dijon mustard (the zesty touch)
- One tablespoon of honey (the subtle sweetness)
- 1/4 cup of olive oil (the silky binder)
- Salt and pepper, to taste

Nutritional Information:

Per serving: Estimated values: 290 calories, 8g protein, 20g carbohydrates, 20g fat, 4g fiber, 13mg cholesterol, 320mg sodium, 400mg potassium.

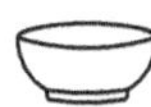

Prep Time: 15 min

Cook Time: 30 min
(for beet roasting)

Serves: 4

Directions

1. **Roasting the Beets:** Preheat your oven to 400°F (200°C). Toss the beet cubes with olive oil, salt, and pepper. Spread them on a baking tray and roast for about 30 minutes or until they are tender and have a caramelized finish. This simple step enhances their deep, natural sweetness and full-bodied flavor, making you feel like a pro in the kitchen.
2. **Prepare the Dressing:** While the beets are in the oven, whisk together the honey, balsamic vinegar, olive oil, and Dijon mustard in a small mixing bowl. Season with salt and pepper to your preference. This dressing will serve as the flavorful link that ties the various elements of the salad together.
3. **Assemble the Salad:** Lay the mixed greens in a large salad bowl as the foundation. Evenly spread the roasted beets, crumbled goat cheese, and toasted walnuts over the greens.
4. **Dress and Mix:** Drizzle the balsamic dressing over the assembled salad before serving. Toss everything gently to ensure the dressing coats the greens and toppings evenly, enhancing the overall flavor with each bite.
5. **Serve Immediately:** Serve the salad immediately to fully enjoy its vibrant flavors and textures, which make it visually and gastronomically appealing.

Summary:

This **Balsamic Beet and Goat Cheese Salad** is a celebration of freshness, blending the robust flavors of roasted beets with the creamy texture of goat cheese and the crunch of walnuts, all brought together by an enthusiastic balsamic dressing. This salad showcases the fresh and simple flavors of garden-fresh ingredients, making it an ideal choice for a refined yet straightforward lunch or a classy side dish at dinner. Enjoy a culinary creation that delights the senses and enriches any meal.

SMOKED SALMON AND AVOCADO ON RYE RECIPE

Ingredients

- 4 slices of dark rye bread (the sturdy foundation)
- 8 ounces of smoked salmon (the flavorful protein)
- 1 ripe avocado, sliced (the smooth texture)
- 1 tablespoon of fresh lemon juice (for freshness and color retention)
- Fresh dill for garnish (the herbal accent)
- Freshly cracked black pepper (for a spicy touch)
- Optional: capers or slices of red onion for added zest

Nutritional Information:

Per serving: Estimated values 220 calories, 4g protein, 24g carbohydrates, 12g fat, 5g fiber, 0mg cholesterol, 0mg sodium, and 200mg potassium.

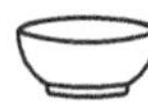  

Prep Time: 10 min   Cook Time: 0 min   Serves: 4

Directions

1. **Preparing the avocado is a breeze.** Cut it into slices and sprinkle with lemon juice to keep it fresh and prevent discoloration.
2. **Assembly:** Place the rye bread slices on a clean surface. Evenly distribute the smoked salmon on each slice. Carefully place avocado slices atop the salmon.
3. **Garnish and Season:** Scatter fresh dill over the assembled layers for an herbal flavor boost. Add capers or red onion for extra zest, and season with black pepper to bring out the flavors if desired.
4. **Serve:** Present immediately to enjoy the blend of hearty, creamy, and zesty flavors.

Summary:

Our **Smoked Salmon and Avocado on Rye** dish is a culinary masterpiece. The salty smoked salmon pairs perfectly with the creamy avocado, all atop a robust rye bread. The result is a sophisticated flavor experience that's perfect for an upscale breakfast, a refined brunch, or a fulfilling light dinner.

MANGO CHICKEN SALAD

Ingredients

- 4 slices of dark rye bread (the sturdy carrier)
- 8 ounces of smoked salmon (the flavor-packed protein)
- 1 avocado, ripe and sliced (the creamy compliment)
- 1 tablespoon of lemon juice (for zest and color preservation)
- Fresh dill for garnishing (the fragrant highlight)
- Ground black pepper freshly cracked (for a subtle warmth)
- Optional: capers or thin slices of red onion for an extra tang

Nutritional Information:

Per serving: Estimated values 290 calories, 18g protein, 20g carbs, 15g fat, 5g fiber, 20mg cholesterol, 760mg sodium, 400mg potassium.

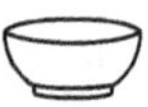

Prep Time: 15 min   Cook Time: 10 min   Serves: 4

Directions

1. **Avocado Preparation:** Slice the avocado and sprinkle it with lemon juice to retain its vivid color and enhance its taste.
2. **Construction:** Place rye bread slices down. Equally, distribute the smoked salmon on each. Neatly arrange avocado slices over the salmon.
3. **Embellishment:** Sprinkle with dill for a herby flair. If desired, incorporate capers or red onion for additional zing. Season with black pepper to fuse the flavors.
4. **Presentation:** Serve promptly to savor the interplay of hearty rye, smooth salmon, and lush avocado.

Summary:

The **Mango Chicken Salad** is an artful medley of sweet, savory, and spicy notes, ideal for any occasion that calls for a light and gratifying meal. Juicy mango and crisp cucumber contrast wonderfully with the robust grilled chicken, all united by a zesty, subtly spicy lime dressing.

Ingredients

- 14 oz firm tofu, drained and cubed (the protein staple)
- 1 tablespoon curry powder (the flavor explosion)
- 1/4 cup plain yogurt or vegan substitute (for added creaminess)
- 1 tablespoon of lemon juice (the citrus spark)
- 1/2 cup grapes, halved (the burst of sweetness)
- 1/2 cup celery, finely diced (the crisp texture)
- 1/4 cup sliced almonds (the added crunch)
- Salt and pepper, to preference (the taste adjusters)
- Fresh cilantro or parsley, finely chopped (for decoration)

Nutritional Information:

Per serving: Estimated values: 200 calories, 12g protein, 15g carbohydrates, 10g fat, 4g fiber, 0mg cholesterol, 300mg sodium, 350mg potassium.

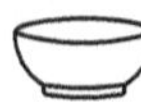  

Prep Time: 15 min

Cook Time: None (additional marinating time)

Serves: 4

Directions

1. **Tofu Marination:** In a mixing bowl, combine the curry powder, yogurt, and lemon juice. Add the tofu cubes and gently stir to coat them. Refrigerate to marinate for at least 30 minutes, enabling the tofu to soak up the flavorful spices fully.
2. **Prepare the Crunchy and Sweet Elements:** As the tofu marinates, ready the grapes, celery, and almonds. These will provide various textures and tastes that enhance the salad experience.
3. **Assemble the Salad:** Once the marination is complete, mix the marinated tofu with the grapes, celery, and almonds. Season with salt and pepper and toss delicately to blend the ingredients while preserving the tofu's integrity.
4. **Garnishing:** Before serving, top the salad with chopped cilantro or parsley for a fresh, herbal accent and a splash of color.
5. **Serving:** Serve the salad chilled. It is an ideal, refreshing dish that packs a good protein punch, suitable for a light meal or a nutritious dinner side.

Summary:

The **Curried Tofu Salad** is a journey of flavors, combining the aromatic warmth of curry with the silky texture of yogurt-enveloped tofu, complemented by the sweet juiciness of grapes and the crispness of celery and almonds. This salad transcends ordinary fare, presenting a nutritious and flavorful choice that invigorates the senses. It's not just a meal; it's an exploration of bold flavors and wholesome ingredients, perfect for those seeking a culinary adventure. Celebrate a dish that is as beneficial to your well-being as it is delightful to your taste buds.

Conclusion: Lunch Made Simple

In this chapter of **"Delicious Diabetic Cookbook for Beginners,"** we've delved into a diverse selection of lunch options. Whether you're enjoying a peaceful meal at home, preparing lunch for work, or needing a quick and satisfying meal, we've got you covered. These recipes offer delicious and nutritious meals that align with your health goals, providing flavors perfect for maintaining a healthy diabetic lifestyle.

From the heartiness of wraps and the freshness of salads to the comforting warmth of soups, these meals ensure that lunchtime is always exciting and never nutritionally compromising.

We've meticulously balanced carbohydrates, protein, and fats in these recipes to help maintain stable blood sugar levels. Each recipe offers a variety of flavors to cater to all tastes and preferences. These simple lunches allow you to enjoy tasty, healthy dishes that align with your wellness goals. Embrace these recipes as your midday fuel, powering a healthy lifestyle with every bite.

Enjoy exploring these simple pleasures that promise satisfaction without stress, keeping your days light, your body energized, and your palate pleased.

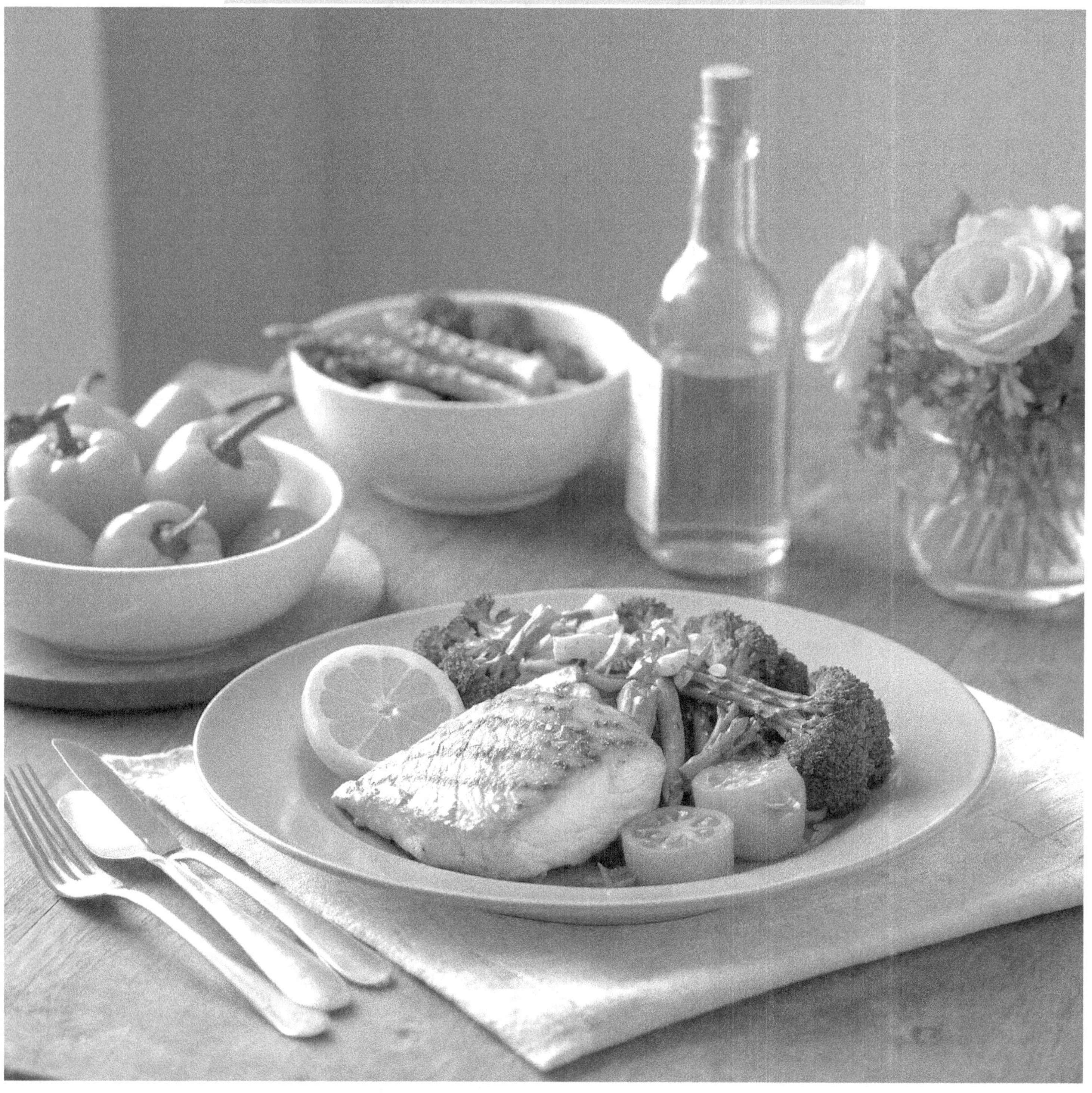

Dinners to Delight: Flavorful dinner recipes that the whole family will enjoy and designed to support blood sugar control without sacrificing taste.

"Dinners to Delight" is a beautifully curated section of the **"Delicious Diabetic Cookbook for Beginners"** that transforms dinner into a delightful experience for the whole family.

Every recipe is crafted to enchant the taste buds and support blood sugar control, which is crucial for managing diabetes. This chapter proves that diabetic-friendly meals can be as diverse and compelling as any other cuisine, breaking the myth that health-focused food must compromise on taste.

These simple and user-friendly recipes ensure that anyone can whip up a healthy and tasty meal any evening. Whether you're looking for a quick weeknight dinner or something special for the weekend, **"Dinners to Delight"** offers options that ensure no one at the table misses out on a fulfilling dining experience. It's a voyage to the core of healthy dining, where each meal is a chance to nurture both body and spirit. **Here's to dinners that promise to be as joyful as they are beneficial, ensuring that every meal is a highlight of the day.**

GARLIC LEMON CHICKEN STIR-FRY

Ingredients

- 1 pound chicken breast, thinly sliced (the primary protein)
- 2 bell peppers (one red, one yellow), sliced (the vibrant elements)
- 3 tablespoons olive oil (used for frying)
- 2 garlic cloves, minced (the taste enhancer)
- Juice and zest of one lemon (the citrusy accent)
- 2 tablespoons soy sauce (the flavor deepener)
- 1 tablespoon of honey (a hint of sweetness)
- Salt and pepper, to preference (basic seasoning)
- Optional: sesame seeds and green onions, chopped

Nutritional Information:

Per serving: Estimated values 290 calories, 18g protein, 20g carbs, 15g fat, 5g fiber, 20mg cholesterol, 760mg sodium, 400mg potassium.

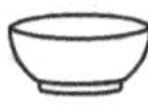  

Prep Time: 15 min   Cook Time: 10   Serves: 4

Directions

1. **Marinate Chicken:** In a bowl, mix the chicken slices with lemon zest, lemon juice, soy sauce, and honey. Season with salt and pepper. Marinate for at least ten minutes to enrich the flavors.
2. **Fry Chicken:** Heat two tablespoons of olive oil over medium-high heat in a large skillet or wok. Cook the marinated chicken (keep the marinade aside) until it's golden and fully cooked, about 5-6 minutes. Remove and set aside.
3. **Sauté Vegetables:** Heat the remaining olive oil in the same skillet. Add the bell peppers and garlic, sautéing until they soften, approximately four minutes.
4. **Mix and Heat:** Add the chicken to the skillet with the vegetables, pouring the saved marinade over it. Cook everything together for two more minutes to blend the flavors.
5. **Presentation:** If using, sprinkle sesame seeds and green onions as garnish. Serve hot, ideally with a side of brown rice or quinoa.

Summary:

The **Garlic Lemon Chicken Stir-Fry** is a delightful concoction that pairs silky chicken with crisp, colorful bell peppers, all tied together with a tangy lemon and subtle sweet garlic sauce. This dish is ideal for a quick weeknight dinner yet elegant enough for entertaining guests. It offers a balanced, nutritious meal that complements a health-oriented lifestyle.

HERB-CRUSTED SALMON

Ingredients

- 4 salmon fillets (6 ounces each, the centerpiece of the meal)
- 2 tablespoons olive oil (for coating)
- 1/4 cup fresh parsley, finely chopped (adds freshness)
- 1/4 cup fresh dill, finely chopped (provides aroma and taste)
- 2 teaspoons of lemon zest (for a citrusy lift)
- 2 garlic cloves, minced (adds robust flavor)
- Salt and pepper, to preference (for seasoning)
- Lemon wedges for garnish

Nutritional Information: Per serving: Estimated values: 310 calories, 34 grams of protein, 1 gram of carbohydrates, 18 grams of fat, no fiber, 90 milligrams of cholesterol, 250 milligrams of sodium, and 450 milligrams of potassium.

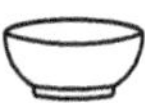  

Prep Time: 10 min   Cook Time: 0 min   Serves: 4

Directions

1. **Oven Preparation:** Heat your oven to 400°F (200°C). Prepare a baking sheet with parchment paper or a light coating of oil.
2. **Herb Mixture Preparation:** In a small bowl, combine parsley, dill, lemon zest, minced garlic, salt, and pepper.
3. **Salmon Preparation:** Arrange the salmon fillets on the baking sheet. Brush each with olive oil.
4. **Apply Herb Mix:** Thickly layer the herb mixture onto each fillet, pressing to ensure it adheres well.
5. **Baking:** Transfer the salmon to the oven and bake for 12 to 15 minutes, or until the fish is thoroughly cooked and easily flakes with a fork.
6. **Presentation:** Serve the baked salmon immediately with lemon wedges for extra flavoring.

Summary:

This **Herb-Crusted Salmon** is a celebration of simple ingredients coming together to create a dish that's as nutritious as it is delicious. The fresh herbs and lemon zest form a crust that not only infuses the salmon with vibrant flavors but also creates a delightful texture contrast to the tender, juicy flesh of the fish. Enjoy a meal that feels like a treat while perfectly fitting into a health-conscious lifestyle. Here's to a dish that's as easy to prepare as it is enjoyable to eat.

BAKED COD WITH OLIVES AND TOMATOES

Ingredients

- 4 cod fillets (6 ounces each, the focus)
- 1 cup of cherry tomatoes halved (adds sweetness)
- 1/2 a cup of pitted Kalamata olives, halved (brings a rich, salty flavor)
- 2 tablespoons capers (adds a tangy element)
- 3 cloves garlic, thinly sliced (flavor enhancer)
- 1/4 cup olive oil (for richness and moisture)
- 1 lemon, sliced
- Fresh basil leaves for garnish
- Salt and pepper, to taste

Nutritional Information:

Per serving: Estimated values: 240 calories, 23g protein, 6g carbohydrates, 14g fat, 2g fiber, 55mg cholesterol, 380mg sodium, 600mg potassium

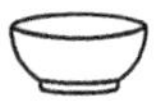  

Prep Time: 10 min   Cook Time: 20 min   Serves: 4

Directions

1. **Preheat the oven:** Heat your oven to 400°F (200°C) and prepare a baking dish.
2. **Prepare the Cod:** Season the cod fillets with salt and pepper. Please place them in a baking dish.
3. **Add Mediterranean Ingredients:** Distribute tomatoes, olives, capers, and garlic around and atop the cod. Drizzle with olive oil.
4. **Bake:** Top the cod with lemon slices. Cook for 15-20 minutes or until the fish flakes easily with a fork.
5. **Garnish and Serve:** Remove from oven, garnish with fresh basil, and serve immediately.

Summary:

Baked Cod with Olives and Tomatoes is a simple yet flavorful dish that brings Mediterranean flair to your table. This dish is ideal for a quick and healthy weeknight meal that doesn't compromise on flavor, providing a delightful dining experience that supports a balanced diet.

Vegetable Lasagna

Ingredients

- 1 zucchini, thinly sliced (introduces a fresh layer)
- 1 eggplant, thinly sliced (provides a substantial texture)
- 1 red bell pepper, sliced (adds color and sweetness)
- 2 cups ricotta cheese (for a creamy texture)
- 1 cup shredded mozzarella cheese (for gooeyness)
- 1/2 cup grated Parmesan cheese (for a salty flavor enhancement)
- 3 cups tomato sauce, homemade or store-bought (serves as a savory base)
- 2 tablespoons of olive oil (used for roasting the vegetables)
- 1 teaspoon of dried oregano (adds herbal notes)
- 1 teaspoon of dried basil (provides sweetness and aroma)
- Salt and pepper, to taste (for seasoning)
- Optional: fresh basil for garnish (for additional freshness)

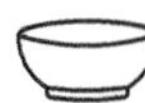  

Prep Time: 20 min   Cook Time: 45 min   Serves: 6

Directions

1. **Roast Vegetables:** Heat your oven to 375°F (190°C). Mix zucchini, eggplant, and bell pepper with olive oil, salt, and pepper. Spread on a baking sheet and roast until tender, about 15 minutes.
2. **Assemble Lasagna:** Start with a layer of tomato sauce in a baking dish. Add a layer of roasted vegetables, spoonful of ricotta cheese, mozzarella, and Parmesan. Repeat the layers, ending with cheese on top.
3. **Baking:** Sprinkle with oregano and basil, then bake for 30 minutes or until the cheese is bubbly and golden.
4. **Rest and Serve:** Let the lasagna cool for 10 minutes to set. Garnish with fresh basil before serving if using.

Nutritional Information:

Per serving: Estimated values: 350 calories, 22g protein, 25g carbohydrates, 20g fat, 6g fiber, 45mg cholesterol, 560mg sodium, 670mg potassium.

Summary:

This **Vegetable Lasagna** transforms a classic comfort food into a vibrant, garden-inspired dish, ideal for family dinners or special occasions. Layers of roasted vegetables combined with rich cheeses and savory tomato sauce create a symphony of flavors that delight the palate while fitting into a health-conscious diet.

THAI BEEF SALAD

Ingredients

- 1 pound beef sirloin, thinly sliced (the main protein)
- 4 cups mixed salad greens (for freshness)
- 1 cucumber, thinly sliced (adds crunch)
- 1 carrot, julienned (for sweetness and color)
- 1/2 red onion, thinly sliced (adds a sharp tang)
- 1/4 cup fresh cilantro, chopped (for a herby touch)
- 1/4 cup fresh mint leaves, chopped (for a refreshing flavor)
- 2 tablespoons roasted peanuts, crushed (for a nutty texture)

For the Dressing:

- 3 tablespoons fish sauce (for umami)
- 2 tablespoons lime juice (for a citrusy zing)
- 1 tablespoon soy sauce (adds depth)
- 2 teaspoons sugar (to balance flavors)
- 1 garlic clove, minced (for a spicy kick)
- 1 red chili, finely chopped (optional, for heat)

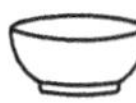  

Prep Time: 15 min   Cook Time: 10 min   Serves: 4

Directions

1. **Cook Beef:** In a skillet over medium-high heat, cook the beef slices for 2-3 minutes per side until browned. Set aside to cool.
2. **To prepare the Dressing, Whisk the** fish sauce, lime juice, soy sauce, sugar, garlic, and chili until the sugar dissolves.
3. **To assemble the Salad, Toss the** mixed greens, cucumber, carrot, onion, cilantro, and mint in a large bowl with the dressing.
4. **Add Beef:** Mix in the beef gently.
5. **Serve:** Plate the salad, topping with crushed peanuts for added crunch.

Nutritional Information:

Per serving: Estimated values: 280 calories, 26g protein, 12g carbohydrates, 16g fat, 3g fiber, 50mg cholesterol, 850mg sodium, 400mg potassium.

Summary:

This **Thai Beef Salad** is a flavorful, colorful dish that combines tender slices of beef with crisp vegetables and a vibrant, zesty Thai dressing. It's a refreshing meal that is both satisfying and light, perfect for a nourishing lunch or a special dinner, and sure to be a delightful addition to any meal plan.

MUSHROOM AND SPINACH RISOTTO

Ingredients

- 1 cup Arborio rice (the foundational starch)
- 2 cups fresh spinach, washed and chopped (adds greenery and nutrients)
- 1 cup fresh mushrooms, sliced (provides earthy tones)
- 1 small onion, finely chopped (the flavor base)
- 2 cloves garlic, minced (enhances the overall taste)
- 4 cups vegetable broth, kept warm (cooking liquid for the rice)
- 1/2 cup white wine (introduces acidity and complexity)
- 1/4 cup grated Parmesan cheese (for richness)
- 2 tablespoons olive oil (used for frying)
- Salt and pepper, to taste (for seasoning)
- Fresh parsley, chopped (for garnish)

Nutritional Information:

Per serving: Estimated values: 310 calories, 9g protein, 47g carbohydrates, 8g fat, 3g fiber, 7mg cholesterol, 460mg sodium, 250mg potassium.

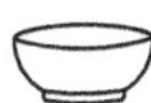  

Prep Time: 10 min   Cook Time: 30 min   Serves: 4

Directions

1. **Sauté Base Ingredients:** Heat olive oil over medium heat in a large pan. Cook the garlic and onion until the onion turns clear.
2. **Cook Mushrooms:** Add the mushrooms and sauté until they brown and release moisture.
3. **Toast Rice:** Add the Arborio rice to the pan, coating it well with oil and lightly toasting it until the edges appear translucent.
4. **Deglaze with Wine:** Add the white wine, stirring continuously until the rice absorbs most of it.
5. **Gradually Add Broth:** Gradually pour in the warm vegetable broth, one ladle at a time, continuously stirring until each ladleful is absorbed before adding the next. This should take about 18-20 minutes.
6. **Incorporate Spinach:** When the risotto is creamy and soft, mix in the spinach and continue cooking until it wilts.
7. **Finish with cheese:** After the heat, mix in the grated Parmesan—season with salt and pepper.
8. **Serve**—dish up the risotto in bowls, garnished with chopped parsley. Enjoy immediately.

Summary:

Mushroom and Spinach Risotto is a comforting and nutritious meal that combines the creamy texture of risotto with the robust flavors of mushrooms and spinach. This dish is a satisfying choice for a cozy dinner, rich in flavors and textures, making it a delightful treat that supports a balanced diet.

TURKEY CHILI

Ingredients

- 1 pound ground turkey (the main protein)
- 1 can (15 ounces) kidney beans, rinsed (adds fiber and texture)
- 1 can (15 ounces) black beans, rinsed (for additional protein and texture)
- 2 cups tomato sauce (the chili base)
- 1 cup diced tomatoes, fresh or canned (for tomato flavor)
- 1 large onion, chopped (adds depth of flavor)
- 1 green bell pepper chopped (provides crunch and color)
- 2 cloves garlic, minced (flavor enhancer)
- 2 tablespoons of chili powder (defines the chili's flavor)
- 1 teaspoon ground cumin (adds a smoky note)
- 1/2 teaspoon red pepper flakes (introduces heat)
- Salt and pepper, to taste (for seasoning)
- Optional garnishes: cilantro, cheese, sour cream, jalapeños

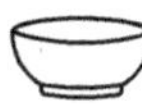  

Prep Time: 15 min   Cook Time: 45 min   Serves: 6

Directions

1. **Brown the Meat:** In a large pot, brown the ground turkey, breaking it up as it cooks.
2. **Sauté Vegetables:** Add onion, bell pepper, and garlic, cooking until softened.
3. **Add Flavors and Tomatoes:** Mix chili powder, cumin, and red pepper flakes. Stir in the tomatoes and tomato sauce.
4. **Simmer:** Incorporate the beans, season with salt and pepper, and let the chili simmer covered on low heat, stirring occasionally.
5. **Finish and Serve:** Adjust seasoning and serve hot with optional garnishes.

Nutritional Information:

Per serving: Estimated values: 295 calories, 23g protein, 34g carbohydrates, 8g fat, 10g fiber, 55mg cholesterol, 720mg sodium, 650mg potassium.

Summary:

Turkey Chili is a hearty, fulfilling dish perfect for warming up on a cold day. It combines lean turkey with beans and spices in a rich tomato base, offering a nutritious meal that satisfies taste and health needs. This chili is ideal for family dinners or meal prep, providing a comforting, flavorful experience.

CAULIFLOWER STEAK

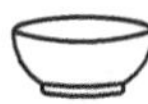  

Ingredients

- 1 large head of cauliflower (the featured vegetable)
- 2 tablespoons olive oil (for roasting)
- 1 teaspoon of garlic powder (adds subtle warmth)
- 1 teaspoon smoked paprika (provides a smoky flavor)
- 1/2 teaspoon ground turmeric (for color and health benefits)
- Salt and pepper, to taste (for seasoning)
- Fresh parsley, chopped (for garnish)

Nutritional Information:

Per serving: Estimated values: 120 calories, 3g protein, 11g carbohydrates, 7g fat, 4g fiber, 0mg cholesterol, 320mg sodium, 430mg potassium.

Prep Time: 10 min   Cook Time: 25 min   Serves: 4

Directions

1. **Preheat Oven:** Set oven to 400°F (200°C) and prepare a baking sheet.
2. **Prepare Cauliflower:** Trim and cut the cauliflower into thick steaks, ensuring each has part of the core.
3. **Season:** Brush with olive oil and season with garlic powder, paprika, turmeric, salt, and pepper.
4. **Roast:** Roast until golden and tender, about 25 minutes, turning once.
5. **Garnish and Serve:** Add parsley for garnish and serve.

Summary:

Cauliflower Steak is an inventive way to enjoy cauliflower, transforming it into a robust, flavorful dish that is a fantastic alternative to traditional steaks. Enhanced with spices and roasted to perfection, it's a visual treat and packed with nutrients, making it a smart choice for those following a healthy diet.

GRILLED SHRIMP TACOS

Ingredients

- 1-pound large shrimp peeled and deveined (succulent and flavorful)
- 8 small corn tortillas (warm and soft)
- 1 avocado, sliced (creamy and rich)
- 1 cup of fresh salsa (zesty and vibrant)
- 1 lime, cut into wedges (for squeezing)
- 2 tablespoons olive oil (for grilling)
- 1 teaspoon of chili powder (for a smoky heat), 1/2 teaspoon garlic powder (subtle flavor boost)
- Salt and pepper, to taste, fresh cilantro, chopped (for garnish)

  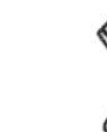

Prep Time: 15 min   Cook Time: 10 min   Serves: 4

Directions

1. **Marinate Shrimp:** In a bowl, mix shrimp with salt, olive oil, chili powder, garlic powder and pepper. Let it marinate for 10 minutes.
2. **Grill Shrimp:** Preheat the grill or grill pan over medium-high heat. Cook shrimp on each side for 2-3 minutes until pink and opaque.
3. **Warm Tortillas:** Encase corn tortillas in a damp cloth and microwave for 30 seconds, or quickly heat on the grill on each side.
4. **Assemble Tacos:** Distribute grilled shrimp onto each tortilla, top with avocado slices, a spoonful of salsa, and a sprinkle of cilantro.
5. **Serve with Lime:** Accompany tacos with lime wedges for added zest when served.

Nutritional Information: Per serving: Estimated values: 310 calories, 24g protein, 35g carbohydrates, 10g fat, 5g fiber, 180mg cholesterol, 320mg sodium, 500mg potassium.

Summary:

Grilled Shrimp Tacos offer a delightful blend of fresh flavors and textures. These tacos feature marinated shrimp grilled to perfection, complemented by creamy avocado and vibrant salsa, all wrapped in warm corn tortillas, perfect for any occasion.

Zucchini Noodle Pad Thai

Ingredients

- 4 medium zucchinis, spiralized into noodles (the fresh base)
- 1/2 pound of shrimp peeled and deveined, or substitute tofu for a vegan option (the primary protein)
- 1 carrot, julienned (adds texture and color)
- 1 red bell pepper, thinly sliced (for sweetness and color)
- 2 green onions, chopped (adds a mild onion flavor)
- 1/4 cup roasted peanuts, chopped (provides crunch)
- 1 egg, lightly beaten (optional; omit for vegan version)
- 2 tablespoons olive oil (used for sautéing)
- Fresh cilantro and lime wedges for garnish (enhances freshness)

For the Sauce:

- 2 tablespoons tamarind paste (the tangy base)
- 2 tablespoons fish sauce or substitute soy sauce for vegan (adds umami)
- 1 tablespoon of rice vinegar (for acidity)
- 2 teaspoons honey or substitute sugar (adds sweetness)
- 1 clove of garlic, minced (enhances flavor)
- 1 red chili, finely chopped, adjust to taste (adds heat)
- 1/2 a teaspoon of ground ginger (a warm note)

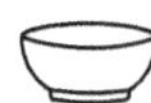  

Prep Time: 20 min   Cook Time: 10 min   Serves: 4

Directions

1. **Prepare the Sauce:** In a small bowl, combine tamarind paste, fish sauce or soy sauce, rice vinegar, honey or sugar substitute, minced garlic, chopped chili, and ginger. Set aside.
2. **Cook Protein:** Heat one tablespoon of olive oil over medium-high heat in a skillet. Cook shrimp or tofu until done, then set aside.
3. **Scramble the Egg:** Use the same skillet to scramble the egg until set, then remove and set aside with the cooked protein.
4. **Sauté Vegetables:** Add another tablespoon of olive oil to the skillet. Sauté carrot and bell pepper until just tender. Stir in zucchini noodles and cook for about two minutes until soft.
5. **Combine and Serve:** Return the protein and egg to the skillet with vegetables. Drizzle the sauce over the mixture, tossing to coat everything evenly. Garnish with green onions, peanuts, cilantro, and lime juice.

Nutritional Information:

Per serving: Estimated values: 250 calories, 18g protein, 20g carbohydrates, 12g fat, 4g fiber, 110mg cholesterol, 620mg sodium, 460mg potassium.

Summary:

This **Zucchini Noodle Pad Thai** reimagines the traditional Thai dish with a healthier twist, using zucchini noodles as a low-carb alternative to rice noodles. The vibrant sauce and fresh vegetables create a flavorful and satisfying dish perfect for a quick dinner or special occasion. Enjoy this lighter version that maintains all the classic flavors of Pad Thai. Plus, it's packed with nutrients and low in calories, making it a smart choice for your health.

PUMPKIN CURRY

Ingredients

- 2 cups pumpkin, peeled and cubed (adds a rich texture and flavor)
- 1 can (14 oz) coconut milk (creamy and aromatic)
- 1 onion, finely chopped (the base flavor)
- 2 cloves garlic, minced (flavor enhancer)
- 1 tablespoon of fresh ginger, grated (adds a zesty warmth)
- 2 tablespoons curry powder (the main spice element)
- 1 teaspoon of turmeric powder (adds color and earthy tones)
- 1 teaspoon cumin seeds (a nutty spice)
- 1/2 a teaspoon of chili flakes (for heat)
- 1 tablespoon olive oil (for sautéing)
- Salt to taste (for seasoning)
- Fresh cilantro, chopped (for garnish)
- Cooked basmati rice to serve (the perfect accompaniment)

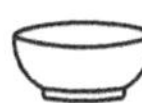  

Prep Time: 15min   Cook Time: 30 min   Serves: 4

Directions

1. **Sauté Aromatics:** Heat olive oil over medium heat in a large pot. Add onion, garlic, ginger, and cumin seeds. Sauté until onion is translucent and spices are aromatic.
2. **Add Spices and Pumpkin:** Stir in curry powder, turmeric, and chili flakes. Add pumpkin and coat well with spices. Pour the coconut milk into the pot and allow it to simmer gently.
3. **Simmer:** Reduce heat and let the curry simmer covered until the pumpkin is tender, about 20-25 minutes.
4. **Final Adjustments:** Season with salt. Adjust consistency with water if needed.
5. **Serve:** Garnish with cilantro. Serve hot and cook basmati rice.

Nutritional Information:

Per serving: Estimated values: 280 calories, 5g protein, 20g carbohydrates, 20g fat, 4g fiber, 0mg cholesterol, 150mg sodium, 600mg potassium.

Summary:

Pumpkin Curry offers a comforting and aromatic experience, perfect for chilly evenings. This curry blends the sweetness of pumpkin with creamy coconut milk and various spices, creating a filling and flavorful dish. It's an ideal option for those seeking a satisfying, health-conscious meal that's easy to prepare and rich in autumnal flavors. Enjoy this warm, spicy curry that's as comforting as it is nutritious. The combination of sweet pumpkin, creamy coconut, and aromatic spices will surely tantalize your taste buds.

Ingredients

- 2 medium eggplants, sliced into half-inch rounds (firm and fresh)
- 2 cups marinara sauce (rich and flavorful)
- 2 cups shredded mozzarella cheese (melty and gooey)
- 1/2 cup grated Parmesan cheese (sharp and salty)
- 1 cup of all-purpose flour (for dredging)
- 2 large eggs, beaten (for egg wash)
- 2 cups breadcrumbs (for crispy coating)
- 1-quarter cup olive oil (for frying)
- Salt and pepper, to taste (seasoning)
- Fresh basil leaves for garnish (adds a fragrant touch)

Nutritional Information:

Per serving: Estimated values: 460 calories, 22g protein, 48g carbohydrates, 22g fat, 7g fiber, 90mg cholesterol, 760mg sodium, 450mg potassium.

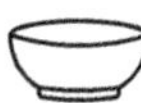

Prep Time: 20 min   Cook Time: 40   Serves: 4

Directions

1. **Prep Eggplant:** Salt the eggplant slices and sit for 20 minutes to draw out moisture. Pat dry.
2. **Dredge and Fry:** Coat each eggplant slice in flour, dip in egg wash, then breadcrumbs. Fry in heated olive oil until golden on each side. Drain on paper towels.
3. **Assemble** Layer fried eggplant in a baking dish with marinara sauce and cheeses. Continue layering until you've used all the ingredients, finishing with a top layer of cheese.
4. **Bake:** Heat oven to 375°F (190°C) and bake for 20-25 minutes until cheese is bubbly and golden.
5. **Garnish and Serve:** Enhance with fresh basil before serving.

Summary:

Eggplant Parmesan is a classic Italian dish featuring layers of golden-fried eggplant smothered in a robust marinara sauce and melted cheeses. This dish, oven-baked until golden, offers a soothing blend of the cheeses' smoothness and the eggplant's soft, succulent texture. It's a hearty and satisfying option perfect for family dinners or special occasions, offering a delightful vegetarian meal as nutritious as it is delicious.

CHICKEN CACCIATORE

Ingredients

- 4 skinless, boneless chicken breasts (lean and tender)
- 1 bell pepper, sliced (colorful and crisp)
- 1 onion, chopped (sweet and robust)
- 2 cups sliced mushrooms (earthy and rich)
- 3 cloves garlic, minced (aromatic and flavorful)
- 2 cups canned diced tomatoes (juicy and vibrant)
- 1/2 cup chicken broth (adds depth)
- 1/4 cup white wine (optional for flavor enhancement)
- 1 teaspoon dried oregano (herby and fragrant)
- 1 teaspoon dried basil (sweet and aromatic)
- Salt and pepper, to taste (for seasoning)
- 2 tablespoons olive oil (for sautéing)
- Fresh parsley, chopped

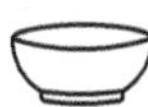  

Prep Time: 20 min   Cook Time: 40 min   Serves: 4

Directions

1. **Sauté Aromatics:** In a skillet, heat olive oil and sauté onion and garlic until translucent.
2. **Brown Chicken:** Add chicken and brown on each side. Remove and set aside.
3. **Cook Vegetables:** In the same skillet, sauté bell pepper and mushrooms until softened.
4. **Simmer:** Return chicken to the skillet with tomatoes, broth, wine, oregano, basil, salt, and pepper. Simmer covered until chicken is cooked through.
5. **Garnish and Serve:** Sprinkle with fresh parsley before serving.

Nutritional Information:

Per serving: Estimated values: 320 calories, 27g protein, 18g carbohydrates, 12g fat, 4g fiber, 70mg cholesterol, 420mg sodium, 650mg potassium.

Summary:

Chicken Cacciatore is a classic Italian dish featuring tender chicken simmered with tomatoes, bell peppers, and mushrooms in a savory broth. This hearty meal fills the kitchen with its rich aromas and offers delicious flavors. Perfect for a family dinner, it provides a comforting and satisfying experience, marrying the sauce's richness with the vegetables' robustness. Enjoy this rustic and flavorful dish that brings the essence of an Italian kitchen to your dining table.

BEEF STIR-FRY WITH BROCCOLI

Ingredients

- 1 pound of lean beef, thinly sliced (like flank steak or sirloin)
- 2 cups broccoli florets (fresh and vibrant)
- 1 bell pepper, sliced (adds color)
- 2 tablespoons soy sauce (for umami flavor)
- 1 tablespoon of fresh ginger, minced (zingy and aromatic)
- 2 cloves garlic, minced (flavorful)
- 2 tablespoons oyster sauce (adds depth)
- 1 tablespoon of sesame oil (for a nutty aroma)
- 1 teaspoon of cornstarch (to subtly thicken the sauce)
- 1/4 cup water
- 2 tablespoons vegetable oil
- Sesame seeds for garnish

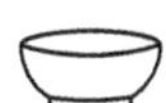  

Prep Time: 15 min   Cook Time: 10 min   Serves: 4

Directions

1. **Prepare the Sauce:** This quick and easy recipe is perfect for a busy evening meal that doesn't compromise taste or health.
2. **Cook the Beef:** Heat oil in a skillet or wok, add beef, and stir-fry until it browns.
3. **Add Vegetables:** Introduce broccoli, bell pepper, ginger, and garlic, and stir-fry until vegetables are tender-crisp.
4. **Combine with Sauce:** Add the prepared sauce to the skillet, cooking until the sauce thickens and coats the ingredients.
5. **Serve:** Sprinkle with sesame seeds and serve right away, preferably over rice or noodles.

Nutritional Information: Per serving: Estimated values: 295 calories, 26g protein, 10g carbohydrates, 18g fat, 3g fiber, 55mg cholesterol, 620mg sodium, 500mg potassium.

Summary:

This **Beef Stir-Fry with Broccoli** is a vibrant and nutritious dish combining tender beef slices with fresh broccoli in a rich, flavorful sauce. Quick and easy to prepare, it's perfect for a busy evening meal that doesn't compromise taste or health. The gingery, garlicky sauce enhances the natural flavors of the beef and vegetables, making each bite a delicious fusion of tastes and textures.

PORTOBELLO MUSHROOM BURGERS

Ingredients

- 4 large portobello mushroom caps stem removed (hearty and meaty)
- 2 tablespoons olive oil (for brushing)
- 1 teaspoon of garlic powder (adds warmth)
- Salt and pepper to taste (for seasoning)
- 4 slices of low-fat mozzarella cheese (light and melty)
- 4 whole wheat burger buns (robust and toasty)
- Lettuce, tomato slices, and red onion (for crisp freshness)
- Optional toppings: mustard, ketchup, or avocado slices

Nutritional Information:

Per serving: Estimated values: 320 calories, 15g protein, 35g carbohydrates, 14g fat, 6g fiber, 15mg cholesterol, 460mg sodium, 550mg potassium.

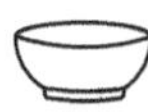  

Prep Time: 15 min   Cook Time: 10 min   Serves: 4

Directions

1. **Prepare the Mushrooms:** Clean the mushroom caps with a damp cloth, brush each olive oil, and season with garlic powder, salt, and pepper.
2. **Grill the Mushrooms:** Heat your grill to medium heat. Cook the mushroom caps gill-side down for about 5 minutes, then flip, add a slice of cheese, and grill for another 5 minutes until the cheese is melted and the mushrooms are tender.
3. **Toast the Buns:** For one or two minutes, toast the buns lightly on the grill.
4. **Assemble the Burgers:** Build the burgers by placing a grilled mushroom on each bun base and adding lettuce, tomato, onion, and other desired toppings.
5. **Serve:** Complete with the top bun and serve immediately for the best flavor.

Summary:
Portobello Mushroom Burgers offers a delectable, vegetarian-friendly alternative to traditional burgers. These burgers feature marinated, grilled portobello caps, a great source of fiber and antioxidants, topped with melted mozzarella and fresh vegetables, providing a variety of essential vitamins and minerals. All of this is nestled within a toasted whole wheat bun, a healthier option than white bread. This meal is satisfying and health-conscious, making it an excellent choice for those looking for a lighter option at a barbecue or family dinner.

LENTIL SOUP WITH KALE

Ingredients

- 1 cup of dried lentils, rinsed (hearty and nutritious)
- 1 bunch of kale stems removed, and leaves chopped (packed with vitamins)
- 1 large onion, diced (sweet base)
- 2 carrots, peeled and diced (adds sweetness)
- 2 celery stalks, diced (provides crunch)
- 3 cloves garlic, minced (flavor enhancer)
- 1 teaspoon of dried thyme (earthy tone)
- 6 cups of low-sodium vegetable broth (for simmering)
- 2 tablespoons olive oil (for sautéing)
- Salt and pepper to taste (for seasoning)
- Optional: red pepper

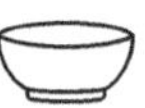  

Prep Time: 10 min   Cook Time: 45 min   Serves: 6

Directions

1. **Sauté Vegetables:** Heat the olive oil over medium heat in a large pot. Cook onion, carrots, and celery until softened, about 5 minutes. Add garlic and thyme, cooking until fragrant, about 1 minute.
2. **Simmer Lentils:** Add lentils and vegetable broth. Bring to a boil, reduce heat, and simmer covered for 30 minutes.
3. **Add Kale:** Mix in the kale and continue simmering until the lentils are tender and the kale has wilted for about 15 minutes. Season with salt, pepper, and optional red pepper flakes.
4. **Adjust Consistency:** Add more water or broth if the soup is too thick.
5. **Serve Warm:** Check seasoning and serve the soup hot, preferably with a slice of crusty whole-grain bread.

Nutritional Information: Per serving: Estimated values: 190 calories, 12g protein, 30g carbohydrates, 4g fat, 12g fiber, 0mg cholesterol, 200mg sodium, 600mg potassium.

Summary:
Our **Lentil Soup with Kale** is more than just a comforting dish. It's a nutritious powerhouse that combines the heartiness of lentils with the health benefits of kale, all seasoned with earthy thyme, perfect for warming up on cool days.

Spaghetti Squash and Meatballs

Ingredients

- 1 large spaghetti squash, approximately four pounds (the main component)
- 1 pound ground turkey (a healthier alternative to traditional beef)
- 1/4 cup breadcrumbs (enhances texture)
- 1/4 cup grated Parmesan cheese (for added flavor)
- 1 large egg (helps bind the meatballs)
- 2 cloves of garlic, minced (adds a robust flavor)
- 1 teaspoon of Italian seasoning (for classic Herby taste)
- 2 cups of low-sodium marinara sauce (rich and full-flavored)
- 1 tablespoon of olive oil (for cooking)
- Salt and pepper, to taste (for seasoning)
- Fresh basil, chopped (for garnish)

Nutritional Information:

Per serving: Estimated values: 350 calories, 28g protein, 35g carbohydrates, 12g fat, 6g fiber, 115mg cholesterol, 480mg sodium, 800mg potassium.

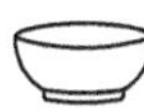

Prep Time: 15 min   Cook Time: 45 min   Serves: 4

Directions

1. **Prepare the Squash:** It's as easy as 1, 2, 3! Set your oven to 400°F (200°C). Cut the spaghetti squash in half lengthwise and discard the seeds. Sprinkle with salt and pepper, coat the inside with olive oil, and lay cut-side down on a baking sheet. Roast until the squash is soft and can be flaked easily with a fork, which should take about 30 to 40 minutes.

2. **Form the Meatballs:** Combine ground turkey, breadcrumbs, grated Parmesan, an egg, minced garlic, Italian seasoning, salt, and pepper in a bowl. Form this mixture into one-inch balls. Warm olive oil in a skillet over medium heat and sauté the meatballs until they are nicely browned. Add marinara sauce and simmer until the meatballs are cooked through, roughly 20 minutes.

3. **Assemble the Dish:** Allow the squash to cool slightly, then shred the inside with a fork to create strands resembling spaghetti. Arrange these squash strands on plates and top them with the meatballs and sauce.

4. **Garnish and Serve:** Add a garnish of fresh basil and serve the dish immediately to enjoy its full flavor.

Summary:

This **Spaghetti Squash and Meatballs** recipe is a unique twist on a beloved Italian classic. The roasted spaghetti squash, a low-carb substitute for pasta, is the star of the show, complemented by savory turkey meatballs in a garlicky marinara sauce. This meal is a flavor explosion, with each bite offering a delightful combination of tastes and textures. It's the perfect dish for those seeking a hearty yet healthy alternative to traditional pasta dishes, and it's sure to impress your family and friends.

Asian Chicken Lettuce Wraps

Ingredients

- 1 pound ground chicken (a lean source of protein)
- 1 head of iceberg lettuce (fresh and crisp)
- 1 carrot, julienned (adds a sweet crunch)
- 1 red bell pepper, thinly sliced (provides a vibrant color)
- 2 green onions, chopped (mild onion flavor)
- 1 tablespoon minced ginger (adds zest)
- 2 cloves garlic, minced (flavor enhancer)
- 2 tablespoons soy sauce (rich in umami)
- 1 tablespoon hoisin sauce (sweet and tangy)
- 1 teaspoon of sesame oil (for a nutty flavor)
- 1/4 cup chopped peanuts (adds crunch)
- Fresh cilantro for garnish

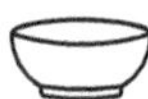  

Prep Time: 20 min   Cook Time: 10 min   Serves: 4

Directions

1. **Prepare Lettuce Cups:** Separate the lettuce leaves, wash, and dry. Set aside as cups for the filling.
2. **Cook Filling:** In a skillet over medium-high heat, brown the ground chicken and drain any excess fat.
3. **Enhance Flavors:** Add ginger and garlic to the chicken, cooking until fragrant. Mix in carrots, bell pepper, green onions, soy sauce, hoisin sauce, and sesame oil, cooking until the vegetables are just tender.
4. **Assemble Wraps:** Spoon the chicken mixture into the lettuce cups. Top with peanuts and cilantro.
5. **Immediate Service:** Serve the wraps immediately, encouraging diners to enjoy fresh and robust flavors.

Nutritional Information: Per serving: Estimated values: 220 calories, 20g protein, 8g carbohydrates, 12g fat, 3g fiber, 65mg cholesterol, 560mg sodium, 350mg potassium.

Summary:

These **Asian Chicken Lettuce Wraps** bring fresh flavors and textures to your table. They feature lean ground chicken infused with aromatic ginger and garlic, wrapped in crisp iceberg lettuce, and garnished with crunchy peanuts and cilantro.

Pesto Pasta with Sun-Dried Tomatoes

Ingredients

- 8 ounces of whole-wheat pasta (nutrient-dense and fibrous)
- 1/2 cup pesto sauce (either homemade or purchased, vibrant and herby)
- 1/3 cup sun-dried tomatoes, chopped (adds a tangy sweetness)
- 1/4 cup grated Parmesan cheese (for a savory, umami richness)
- 1 tablespoon of olive oil (enhances gloss and flavor)
- Salt and pepper to your taste (for seasoning)
- Fresh basil leaves for decoration

Nutritional Information:

Per serving: 320 calories, 10g protein, 40g carbohydrates, 14g fat, 6g fiber, 4mg cholesterol, 380mg sodium, 300mg potassium.

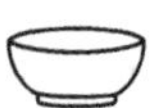  

Prep Time: 10 min   Cook Time: 15 min   Serves: 4

Directions

1. **Cook the Pasta:** Start by boiling a large pot of salted water. Cook the whole-wheat pasta until it reaches al dente consistency, as per the instructions on the package. Drain and set aside.
2. **Mix the Ingredients:** Put the warm pasta into a large bowl and stir it with the pesto sauce to coat each noodle thoroughly. Then, add the chopped sun-dried tomatoes and combine everything nicely.
3. **Incorporate the Cheese:** Sprinkle the grated Parmesan cheese over the pasta, tossing it to distribute the cheese evenly throughout.
4. **Finish and Serve:** Gently sprinkle olive oil over the pasta, add salt and pepper to your taste, and serve the dish while it's still warm. Add fresh basil leaves as a garnish to enhance the freshness.
5. **Optional Enhancements:** Consider adding grilled chicken breast or chickpeas to the dish for added protein.

Summary:

Pesto Pasta with Sun-Dried Tomatoes is a hearty yet refreshing dish that beautifully marries the robust flavors of pesto and the distinct tang of sun-dried tomatoes with wholesome whole-wheat pasta. Finished with a layer of melted Parmesan cheese and adorned with fresh basil for garnish, an ideal quick dinner that does not compromise health or flavor.

BUTTERNUT SQUASH RISOTTO

Ingredients

- 1 medium butternut squash (approximately two cups), peeled and cubed (sweet and earthy)
- 1 tablespoon olive oil (for sautéing and roasting)
- 4 cups vegetable broth (rich and savory base)
- 1 small onion, finely chopped (adds a mild, sweet flavor)
- 1 cup Arborio rice (creamy and starchy, perfect for risotto)
- 1/2 cup dry white wine (adds acidity and depth)
- 1/2 cup grated Parmesan cheese (provides a salty, umami richness)
- 2 tablespoons unsalted butter (for creaminess and richness)
- Salt and freshly ground black pepper, as needed, to enhance flavor.
- Fresh sage leaves for garnish (aromatic and slightly peppery)

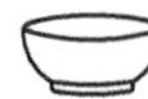

Prep Time: 15 min   Cook Time: 30 min   Serves: 4

Directions

1. **Roast the Squash:** Heat your oven to 425°F (220°C). Brush the butternut squash cubes with olive oil and sprinkle them with salt and pepper. Spread them on a baking sheet and roast until they are tender and golden about 25 minutes.
2. **Warm the Broth:** Keep the vegetable broth heated in a saucepan over low heat.
3. **Sauté Onions:** In a large skillet, melt the butter over medium heat and cook the onion until it becomes translucent. Add the Arborio rice, stirring until the grains are well-coated and start to look slightly translucent at the edges.
4. **Deglaze with Wine:** Pour in the white wine and stir continuously until it has mostly evaporated.
5. **Cook the Rice:** Gradually add the hot broth one ladle at a time, stirring often. Wait until each addition is almost fully absorbed before adding the next until the rice is creamy and al dente, about 20 minutes.
6. **Finish the Dish:** Mix in the roasted butternut squash and Parmesan cheese. Add more butter if desired and adjust the seasoning with salt and pepper.
7. **Serve:** Garnish with fresh sage leaves and serve warm.

Nutritional Information:

Per serving: Estimated values: 410 calories, 9g protein, 58g carbohydrates, 14g fat, 5g fiber, 20mg cholesterol, 630mg sodium, 450mg potassium.

Summary:

Butternut Squash Risotto marries roasted butternut squash's sweet, nutty flavor with creamy, cheesy risotto, creating a rich and comforting dish. This recipe offers a luxurious texture and earthy flavors enhanced by fresh sage, making it perfect for a cozy night or special occasion. It's a warm, inviting dish that combines simple ingredients for a gourmet experience.

TOFU AND VEGETABLE STIR-FRY

Ingredients

- 14 ounces of firm tofu drained and cubed (primary protein source)
- 2 cups broccoli florets (adds crunch and color)
- 1 red bell pepper, sliced (brings sweetness and vibrancy)
- 1 carrot, julienned (adds a slight sweetness)
- 1 zucchini, sliced (mild and satisfying)
- 2 tablespoons soy sauce (enhances umami flavors)
- 1 tablespoon of sesame oil (provides a nutty aroma)
- 1 teaspoon of cornstarch (thickens the sauce)
- ½ a cup of vegetable broth (used for cooking and flavor)
- 2 garlic cloves, minced (foundation of flavor)
- 1 tablespoon of fresh ginger, minced (spicy and warm)
- 2 green onions, chopped (adds a sharp bite)
- Sesame seeds for garnish

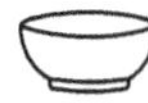  

Prep Time: 15 min   Cook Time: 10 min   Serves: 4

Directions

1. **Prepare Tofu:** Press the tofu to expel excess water, then cube. Lightly fry in a non-stick pan until golden brown. Set aside.
2. **Cook Vegetables:** In the same pan, heat sesame oil and sauté garlic and ginger until aromatic. Add broccoli, bell pepper, carrot, and zucchini. Stir-fry until vibrant and tender-crisp.
3. **Create Sauce:** In a bowl, mix soy sauce, vegetable broth, and cornstarch. Add this mixture to the vegetables in the skillet, stirring continuously until the sauce thickens.
4. **Combine Ingredients:** Return the tofu to the skillet, stirring thoroughly to coat all ingredients evenly with the sauce. Continue to cook for a few more minutes to warm the tofu.
5. **Serve:** Sprinkle with sesame seeds and green onions. Serve hot, preferably over a bed of steamed rice or quinoa.

Nutritional Information: Per serving: Estimated values: 175 calories, 12g protein, 15g carbohydrates, 9g fat, 4g fiber, 0mg cholesterol, 480mg sodium, 350mg potassium.

Summary:

This **Tofu and Vegetable Stir-Fry** is a colorful and nutritious dish, perfect for a quick and healthy meal. It combines the hearty texture of tofu with fresh, crisp vegetables, all brought together by a savory soy sauce-based glaze.

PORK TENDERLOIN WITH APPLES

Ingredients

- 1 pork tenderloin (about 1 to 1.5 pounds) (lean and tender)
- 3 medium apples, cored and sliced (such as Gala or Granny Smith, add a sweet tartness)
- 1 small onion, thinly sliced (enhances flavor)
- 2 tablespoons honey (natural sweetness)
- 2 tablespoons apple cider vinegar (adds a tangy kick)
- 1 teaspoon of ground cinnamon (spicy warmth)
- 1/4 teaspoon ground nutmeg (subtle spice)
- Salt and freshly ground black pepper, according to your preference (for seasoning)
- 2 tablespoons olive oil (for cooking)
- Fresh thyme sprigs (for garnish) (aromatic touch)

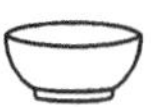  

Prep Time: 20 min   Cook Time: 90 min   Serves: 4

Directions

1. **Preheat Oven:** Set to 375°F (190°C).
2. **Season Pork:** Rub the pork tenderloin with salt and pepper. Sear in an oven-safe skillet with hot olive oil until golden.
3. **Cook Apples and Onions:** Reduce heat, add more oil, and sauté apples and onions. Mix in honey, vinegar, cinnamon, and nutmeg, cooking until apples soften.
4. **Roast:** Return pork to the skillet, surrounding it with the apple mixture, and roast in the oven for 20-25 minutes or until properly cooked.
5. **Serve:** Let the pork rest before slicing. Serve with the apple mixture and garnished with thyme.

Nutritional Information: **Per serving**: Estimated values: Estimated values: 310 calories, 24g protein, 27g carbohydrates, 12g fat, 4g fiber, 75mg cholesterol, 220mg sodium, 650mg potassium.   **Summary:**

Pork Tenderloin with Apples is a dish that tantalizes the senses. The succulent pork tenderloin perfectly complements the sweet and tangy apple mixture, creating a symphony of flavors. Classic spices make the dish ideal for a cozy family dinner.

ROAST BEEF AND VEGETABLES

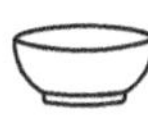

Ingredients

- 2 pounds of beef roast (choose a lean cut like sirloin or round roast for best results)
- 2 carrots, peeled and sliced (adds sweetness and vibrant color)
- 2 parsnips, peeled and sliced (provide an earthy sweetness)
- 1 pound of tiny potatoes halved (brings heartiness to the dish)
- 1 onion, quartered (deepens the savory flavor)
- 3 cloves of garlic minced (intensifies flavors)
- 2 tablespoons of olive oil (used for roasting)
- Salt and pepper, according to taste, 2 sprigs of fresh rosemary

Prep Time: 20 min   Cook Time: 60 min   Serves: 4

Directions

1. **Prepare Vegetables:** In a large roasting pan, combine carrots, parsnips, potatoes, onion, garlic, olive oil, salt, pepper, and rosemary. Toss to coat.
2. **Season and Arrange Beef:** Liberally season the beef roast with salt and pepper. Place it at the center of the roasting pan, surrounded by the seasoned vegetables.
3. **Roasting:** Set your oven to 375°F (190°C). Cook the beef and vegetables for about 60 minutes, or until the meat is cooked to your liking and the vegetables are soft and caramelized.
4. **Resting and Serving:** After removing the beef from the oven, let it sit for 10 minutes. Then, cut it into slices and serve alongside the roasted vegetables.
5. **Additional Garnish:** Optionally, add more fresh rosemary for garnish.

Nutritional Information:

Per serving: Estimated values: 450 calories, 35g protein, 30g carbohydrates, 22g fat, 6g fiber, 90mg cholesterol, 600mg sodium, 800mg potassium.

Summary:

Roast Beef and Vegetables is a classic, comforting meal perfect for family dinners or special occasions. This dish features tender, slow-roasted beef surrounded by a medley of sweet and earthy vegetables, all infused with the flavors of garlic and rosemary.

GRILLED CHICKEN CAESAR SALAD

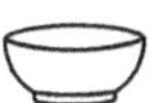

Ingredients

- 4 boneless, skinless chicken breasts (lean and tender)
- 2 heads of romaine lettuce, washed and chopped (crisp and fresh)
- 1 cup of low-fat Caesar dressing (creamy and flavorful)
- 1/2 cup grated Parmesan cheese (adds a salty, umami richness)
- 1 cup of whole-grain croutons (crunchy and hearty)
- 2 tablespoons of olive oil (for grilling the chicken)
- Salt and freshly ground black pepper, to taste (for seasoning)
- Lemon wedges for garnish (adds a fresh, zesty finish)

Prep Time: 15 min   Cook Time: 10 min   Serves: 4

Directions

1. **Preheat Grill:** Prepare your grill for medium-high heat. Brush the chicken breasts with olive oil and season with salt and pepper.
2. **Grill Chicken:** Cook the chicken on the grill for about 5 minutes per side or until fully cooked and the juices clear. Let the chicken rest briefly, then slice thinly.
3. **Assemble the Salad:** In a spacious bowl, mix the chopped romaine lettuce thoroughly with the Caesar dressing until evenly coated. Add the sliced chicken and croutons, and sprinkle with Parmesan cheese.
4. **Serve:** Portion the salad onto plates, garnishing each with lemon wedges. Serve promptly to maintain freshness and texture.

Nutritional Information: Per serving: Estimated values 350 calories, 38g protein, 12g carbohydrates, 18g fat, 3g fiber, 75mg cholesterol, 580mg sodium, 350mg potassium.

Summary:

Grilled Chicken Caesar Salad is a timeless creation that marries succulent grilled chicken with fresh, crisp romaine lettuce, all enhanced by a smooth Caesar dressing. Perfect for a light dinner or a nutritious lunch.

VEGETARIAN CHILI

Ingredients

- 1 can of black beans, drained and rinsed (rich in fiber)
- 1 can of kidney beans, drained and rinsed (contributes to hearty texture)
- 1 can of garbanzo beans, drained and rinsed (excellent source of protein)
- 2 large bell peppers (one red, one green), diced (for a colorful mix)
- 1 large onion, diced (adds a robust flavor)
- 2 zucchinis, diced (for a mild, earthy touch)
- 1 can of corn, drained (sweet kernels)
- 2 cans of diced tomatoes (base of the chili)
- 3 cloves garlic, minced (flavor enhancer)
- 2 tablespoons olive oil (for sautéing)
- 2 tablespoons chili powder (spicy depth)
- 1 tablespoon of cumin (earthy spice)
- 1 teaspoon of smoked paprika (smoky flavor)
- Salt and black pepper to taste (seasoning)
- Fresh cilantro, chopped (for garnish) (herbal freshness)
- Optional: shredded cheddar cheese (for topping) (adds creaminess)

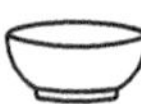  

Prep Time: 20 min   Cook Time: 45 min   Serves: 6

Directions

1. **Sauté Vegetables:** Heat olive oil over medium heat in a large pot. Cook the onion, garlic, and bell peppers until softened, about 5 minutes.
2. **Add Spices:** Incorporate chili powder, cumin, and smoked paprika, cooking until aromatic, about one minute.
3. **Combine Ingredients:** Introduce diced tomatoes, all beans, zucchini, and corn to the pot. Season with salt and pepper.
4. **Simmer:** Lower heat, cover, and simmer for 40 minutes, stirring occasionally.
5. **Serve:** Adjust seasoning, garnish with cilantro and cheese if using, and serve hot.

Nutritional Information:

Per serving: Estimated values: 290 calories, 16g protein, 54g carbohydrates, 5g fat, 15g fiber, 0mg cholesterol, 480mg sodium, 950mg potassium.

Summary:

This **Vegetarian Chili** is not just a robust and hearty dish perfect for warming up on a cold day. It's also a nutritional powerhouse. Packed with three types of beans and various vegetables, it's a filling and flavorful meal that's also rich in fiber and protein. The rich spices add a delightful complexity that makes this chili comforting and irresistibly tasty. It's ideal for anyone seeking a meat-free option that still satisfies the craving for a thick, spicy stew.

GARLIC BUTTER BAKED SALMON

Ingredients

- Four 6-ounce salmon fillets (Four portions of delicious fish)
- 4 tablespoons melted unsalted butter (smooth, golden goodness)
- 3 cloves garlic (finely minced aromatic delight)
- 1 tablespoon of lemon juice
- 1 teaspoon of dried parsley (herbaceous flavor)
- Salt and black pepper (to taste)
- Lemon slices

Nutritional Information:

Per serving: Estimated values: Estimated values: 295 calories, 23g protein, 0g carbohydrates, 22g fat, 0g fiber, 75mg cholesterol, 125mg sodium, 500mg potassium.

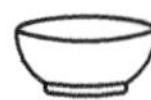  

Prep Time: 10 min   Cook Time: 20 min   Serves: 4

Directions

1. **Preheat Oven:** Preheat your oven to 375°F (190°C). Line a baking sheet with aluminum foil and lightly coat it with cooking spray.
2. **Mix Garlic Butter:** Combine melted butter, garlic, lemon juice, and parsley in a small bowl. Season with salt and pepper.
3. **Prepare Salmon:** Arrange fillets on the prepared sheet. Generously apply the garlic butter mixture with a brush.
4. **Bake:** Place in the oven for 15-20 minutes or until salmon is thoroughly cooked and flakes easily.
5. **Serve:** Enhance with lemon slices and additional parsley if desired. Serve hot.

Summary:

Garlic Butter Baked Salmon is a sumptuous dish that marries the richness of garlic butter with the tenderness of salmon, enhanced by a hint of lemon. It combines simple ingredients for a flavorful experience quick yet elegant dinner option.

ROASTED TURKEY BREAST WITH HERB VEGETABLES

Ingredients

- 2 pounds of turkey breast (bone-in, skin-on for maximum flavor)
- 2 cups of carrots (peeled and sliced, adding sweetness and vibrant color)
- 2 cups of Brussels sprouts (halved for a nutty and earthy texture)
- 2 cups of sweet potatoes (peeled and cubed for heartiness)
- 3 tablespoons of olive oil
- 2 teaspoons of garlic powder
- 2 teaspoons of dried rosemary
- 2 teaspoons of dried thyme
- Salt and pepper
- Fresh parsley

Nutritional Information:

Per serving: 450 calories, 35g protein, 35g carbohydrates, 20g fat, 7g fiber, 85mg cholesterol, 300mg sodium, 900mg potassium.

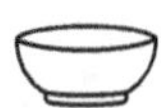  

Prep Time: 20 min   Cook Time: 60 min   Serves: 4

Directions

1. **Preheat and Prepare**: Preheat your oven to 375°F (190°C) and prepare a large baking tray with parchment paper.
2. **Season the Turkey**: Massage one tablespoon of olive oil into the breast. Season liberally with salt, pepper, garlic powder, rosemary, and thyme. Position in the center of the prepared tray.
3. **Prepare Vegetables**: In the remaining olive oil, mix the carrots, Brussels sprouts, and sweet potatoes. Season with salt, pepper, and additional herbs as preferred. Spread these vegetables around the turkey on the tray.
4. **Roast**: Place the tray in the oven and roast for approximately 60 minutes, or until the turkey's internal temperature hits 165°F (74°C) and the vegetables become tender and have caramelized.
5. **Serve**: Let the turkey rest for 10 minutes before slicing. Arrange slices alongside the herb-infused vegetables, topped with fresh parsley for garnish.

Summary:

The **Roasted Turkey Breast** with Herb Vegetables recipe is a sensory delight, perfect for festive occasions or a comforting family meal. As the turkey roasts, the rich blend of herbs fills the air with savory aromas, building anticipation for the juicy, flavorful experience to come.

TANGY TOMATO BRUSCHETTA

Ingredients

- 1 cup chopped ripe tomatoes (fresh and juicy)
- 1/4 cup chopped red onion (crisp and pungent)
- 1/4 cup chopped fresh basil (aromatic and green)
- 2 tablespoons balsamic vinegar (rich and tangy)
- 1 tablespoon olive oil (smooth and fruity)
- Salt and pepper to taste (for seasoning)
- 4 slices whole-grain baguette, toasted (hearty and rustic)

Nutritional Information:

Per serving: 120 calories, 3g protein, 18g carbohydrates, 5g fat, 3g fiber, 0mg cholesterol, 150mg sodium, 200mg potassium.

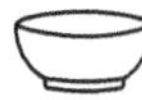  

Prep Time: 10 min   Cook Time: 0 min   Serves: 4

Directions

1. **Combine:** In a mixing bowl, toss the tomatoes, red onion, basil, balsamic vinegar, and olive oil—season with salt and pepper to taste.
2. **Assemble:** Spoon the tomato mixture generously over the toasted baguette slices.
3. **Serve:** Enjoy immediately, savoring the vibrant flavors and fresh textures.

Summary:

Tangy Tomato Bruschetta offers fresh flavors, combining ripe tomatoes with aromatic basil and a tangy balsamic kick. Perfect for a light snack or a starter, this dish brings the essence of Italian cuisine to your table, making it healthy and delightfully satisfying.

CREAMY AVOCADO SALSA

Ingredients

- 2 ripe avocados, diced (creamy and lush)
- 1 cup cherry tomatoes, halved (sweet and vibrant)
- 1/4 cup finely chopped red onion (sharp and colorful)
- 1 jalapeno, seeded and minced (for a mild kick)
- Juice of 1 lime (bright and zesty)
- Salt and pepper to taste (for seasoning)
- A handful of cilantros, chopped (fresh and herby)

Nutritional Information:

Per serving: 160 calories, 3g protein, 10g carbohydrates, 13g fat, 5g fiber, 0mg cholesterol, 200mg sodium, 400mg potassium.

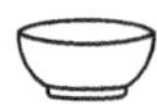  

Prep Time: 10 min   Cook Time: 0 min   Serves: 4

Directions

1. **Mix:** In a bowl, combine the diced avocados, cherry tomatoes, red onion, jalapeno, and lime juice. Gently toss to mix well without mashing the avocados.
2. **Flavor:** Season with salt and pepper, adjusting according to your taste.
3. **Garnish:** Sprinkle with chopped cilantro for an added fresh touch.
4. **Serve:** Offer this creamy salsa with whole-grain tortilla chips or a topping for grilled chicken or fish.

Summary:

Creamy Avocado Salsa blends the smoothness of avocados with the tang of lime and the crunch of fresh vegetables. Its vibrant colors make it not only a joy to look at but also a delight to eat, making it a perfect addition to any meal or as a stand-alone snack.

SPICY TOFU AND VEGETABLE CURRY

Ingredients

- 4 large bell peppers (any color, halved and seeded for a colorful and customizable base)
- 1 cup of cooked quinoa (provides a nutty texture and is rich in protein)
- 1 15-ounce can of black beans (rinsed and drained adds a fiber-rich component to the dish)
- 1 cup of corn kernels (adds a sweet crunch, fresh or frozen)
- 1/2 cup onion (finely chopped for a foundational flavor)
- 1 teaspoon of garlic powder (provides a robust garlic flavor without the hassle)
- 1 teaspoon cumin (for a warm, earthy note)
- 1/2 teaspoon chili powder (adds a mild spice)
- 1/2 cup low-sodium vegetable broth (helps to steam and cook the peppers)
- 1 cup shredded cheddar cheese (for a creamy, melty texture)
- Salt and pepper
- Fresh cilantro (chopped)

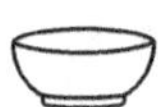  

Prep Time: 15 min	Cook Time: 30 min	Serves: 4

Directions

1. **Prepare Tofu:** Press tofu to remove excess water, cube, and fry in a pan with one tablespoon oil until golden. Set aside.
2. **Sauté Vegetables:** Use the remaining oil to sauté onion, garlic, ginger, carrots, bell peppers, and zucchini until tender.
3. **Add spices and simmer:** Sprinkle with curry powder, cumin, and turmeric, and cook briefly to release flavors. Stir in tomatoes and coconut milk, simmer, then add the tofu.
4. **Combine and Serve:** Continue to simmer gently, season to taste. Serve the curry over cooked rice.

Nutritional Information:

Per serving: 410 calories, 18g protein, 45g carbohydrates, 20g fat, 6g fiber, 0mg cholesterol, 480mg sodium, 800mg potassium.

Summary:

Spicy Tofu and Vegetable Curry is not just a flavorful meal but also a health powerhouse. This curry, packed with colorful vegetables and protein-rich tofu, is a perfect choice for those seeking a hearty yet healthy vegan option. With a rich, tangy sauce and a burst of freshness from the cilantro garnish, this curry is not only satisfying but also a nutrient-dense meal, ideal for a comforting dinner any day of the week.

As we conclude the diverse and flavorful 'Dinners to Delight' chapter of the **"Delicious Diabetic Cookbook for Beginners,"** it's evident that we've catered to a wide range of tastes and preferences. From succulent seafood dishes to hearty vegetarian options, each recipe is a testament to our commitment to providing various diabetes-friendly meals. We believe that managing diabetes or cooking for a loved one who has diabetes should never mean sacrificing taste or variety. Each dish, lovingly created to be both nourishing and satisfying, promises a delightful dinner experience that brings comfort and joy to your table. Whether you're seeking the warmth of a slow-cooked stew or the zest of an exotic stir-fry, this collection transforms your evening meals into a celebration of flavors that all family members, regardless of their dietary needs, can enjoy.

Each recipe in this cookbook is a gateway to new flavors and culinary experiences. Embrace them as opportunities to create memorable moments around your dinner table filled with excitement and curiosity.

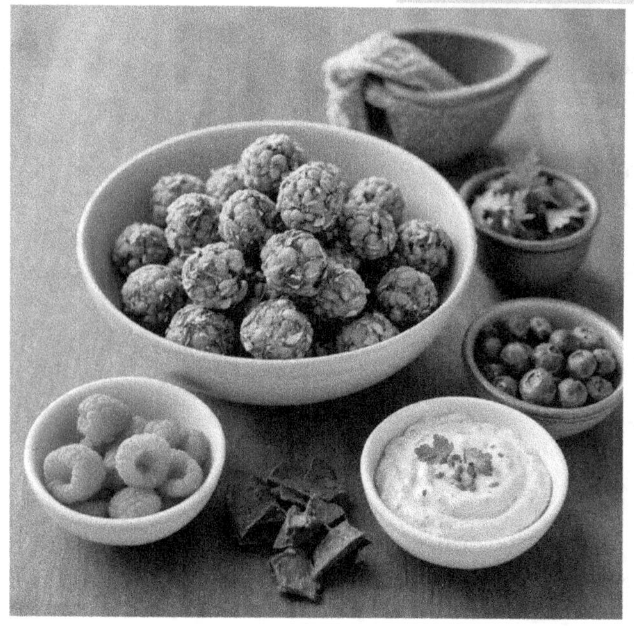

In the "**Snack Smart**" section of the "**Delicious Diabetic Cookbook for Beginners,**" you'll discover various nutritious snack ideas designed to satisfy mid-day cravings without causing spikes in blood sugar levels.

This chapter shows that snacking can be delicious and friendly from a delightful and guilt-free indulgence. From crunchy vegetable chips paired with savory dips to sweet, guilt-free treats and protein-packed bites, each snack is thoughtfully crafted to balance flavors and nutrients, offering a variety of exciting possibilities for your snacking journey, leaving you feeling indulged and satisfied, maintaining a healthy lifestyle and empower you to indulge in flavors that excite the palate. The recipes are designed to be simple, quick to prepare, and use readily available ingredients, ensuring you're always just a few steps away from a satisfying snack.

Whether you need a quick pick-me-up between meals or a healthy option to tide you over until dinner, the "**Snack Smart**" chapter offers creative and tasty solutions that keep your taste buds and blood sugar in check. **Embrace these wholesome alternatives as your go-to resource for snacking without compromise.**

CHIA SEED PUDDING WITH MIXED BERRIES

Ingredients

- 1/4 cup chia seeds (for a gelatinous texture and omega-3s)
- 1 cup of unsweetened almond milk (provides a nutty flavor and creamy base)
- 1 tablespoon of honey or maple syrup (for natural sweetness)
- 1/2 teaspoon vanilla extract (enhances aroma and depth of flavor)
- 1 cup mixed berries (like strawberries, blueberries, and raspberries for antioxidants and vibrant color)
- A pinch of salt (enhances flavors)

Nutritional Information:

Per serving: 130 calories, 4g protein, 15g carbohydrates, 5g fat, 7g fiber, 0mg cholesterol, 80mg sodium, 200mg potassium.

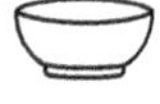  

Prep Time: 10 min

Cook Time: 0 min

Serves: 4

Refrigeration Time: at least 4 hours or overnight

Directions

1. **Blend Ingredients:** In a bowl, blend chia seeds, almond milk, honey or maple syrup, vanilla extract, and a touch of salt.
2. **Rest and Thicken:** Seal the bowl and chill in the refrigerator for at least four hours, ideally overnight, to let the chia seeds expand and achieve a consistency of pudding.
3. **Prepare Berries:** Rinse the mixed berries and slice any larger berries before serving.
4. **Serve:** Distribute the thickened chia pudding into bowls or glasses, topping each with fresh berries.
5. **Garnish:** Optionally, enhance with extra honey or maple syrup and sprinkle a few whole chia seeds or mint leaves for added flair.

Summary:

Chia Seed Pudding with Mixed Berries is a healthful, refreshing treat that's incredibly simple to prepare. This pudding, loaded with omega-3 fatty acids and essential nutrients from the chia seeds and a vibrant mix of berries, is perfect as a breakfast, snack, or light dessert. It satisfies sweet cravings with natural ingredients, making health-conscious individuals feel at ease.

Spiced Chickpea Crunchies

Ingredients

- 1 can (15 ounces) chickpeas, drained and rinsed (offers a protein-rich base)
- 1 tablespoon of olive oil (ensures crispiness)
- ½ teaspoon ground cumin (provides a warm, earthy flavor)
- ½ teaspoon chili powder (adds a touch of heat)
- 1/4 teaspoon salt (enhances flavor)
- 1/4 teaspoon black pepper (provides a slight kick)

Nutritional Information

Per serving: 180 calories, 6g protein, 20g carbohydrates, 7g fat, 6g fiber, 0mg cholesterol, 300mg sodium, 250mg potassium.

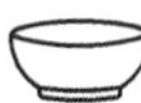  

Prep Time: 10 min | Cook Time: 40 min | Serves: 4

Directions

1. **Preheat oven and prepare chickpeas:** Set oven to 400°F (200°C). Dry the chickpeas thoroughly with paper towels to remove moisture—this step is crucial for maximum crunchiness.
2. **Season:** Toss chickpeas with olive oil, cumin, chili powder, salt, and pepper until evenly coated.
3. **Roast:** Spread the chickpeas in a single layer on a baking sheet. Roast in the oven for around 35-40 minutes, stirring every 10 minutes, until they turn golden brown and crisp.
4. **Cool and Serve:** Let chickpeas cool slightly to enhance their crunchiness. Once completely cooled, they can be enjoyed warm or stored in an airtight container.

Summary:

We are looking for a snack that's both healthy and delicious. Our **Spiced Chickpea Crunchies** are the perfect choice. Bursting with flavor and offering an ideal crunch, these chickpeas are a nutritious snack that satisfies without guilt. They can also contribute a crunchy texture to salads or act as an exciting feature at any event.

Cucumber Rolls with Hummus

Ingredients

- 2 large English cucumbers, thinly sliced lengthwise (provide crisp wraps)
- 1 cup of hummus (creamy and flavorful)
- 1/4 cup of roasted red peppers, finely chopped (adds color and sweetness)
- 1 tablespoon of fresh dill, chopped (for a fresh, herbal note)
- Add salt and pepper to your taste (for seasoning)

Nutritional Information:

Per serving: 150 calories, 6g protein, 13g carbohydrates, 9g fat, 5g fiber, 0mg cholesterol, 300mg sodium, 200mg potassium.

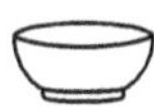  

Prep Time: 15 min | Cook Time: 0 min | Serves: 4

Directions

1. **Prepare Cucumbers:** Slice the cucumbers into thin strips using a mandoline or a sharp knife. Place the strips on paper towels to absorb any excess moisture.
2. **Add Filling:** Evenly spread hummus on each cucumber strip and sprinkle with roasted red peppers and dill.
3. **Roll Them Up:** Carefully roll each strip into a tight spiral with the hummus on the inside. Secure with a toothpick if needed.
4. **Season and Serve:** Adjust the seasoning with salt and pepper. Serve immediately or chill in the refrigerator for about an hour to enhance the flavors.

Summary:

These **Cucumber Rolls with Hummus** blend the crisp freshness of cucumber with the rich, creamy texture of hummus, enhanced by the zesty taste of roasted red peppers and dill. They are perfect as a light, refreshing snack or an elegant gathering appetizer. This simple yet sophisticated dish is visually appealing and delicious, providing a healthy option that satisfies both the palate and nutritional needs.

Nutty Cocoa Energy Balls

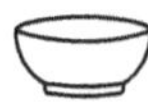  

Ingredients

- 1 cup of Medjool dates, pitted (natural sweetness and sticky texture)
- ½ cup of mixed nuts (almonds, walnuts, pecans for crunch and protein)
- 2 tablespoons of cocoa powder (rich chocolate flavor)
- 1 tablespoon of chia seeds (adds omega-3s and fiber)
- 1 teaspoon of vanilla extract (enhances flavor)
- A pinch of salt (flavor enhancer)

Nutritional Information:

Per serving: 220 calories, 5g protein, 30g carbohydrates, 11g fat, 6g fiber, 0mg cholesterol, 20mg sodium, 300mg potassium.

Prep Time: 10 min · Cook Time: 0 min · Serves: 4

Directions

1. **Mix Base:** In a food processor, blend the dates, nuts, cocoa powder, chia seeds, vanilla extract, and a pinch of salt until the mixture combines and sticks together.
2. **Shape the Balls:** Take tablespoon-sized scoops of the mixture and roll them into balls between your hands.
3. **Refrigerate:** Set the energy balls on a parchment-covered baking sheet and refrigerate for approximately 30 minutes to allow them to firm up.
4. **Serving and Storage:** Serve the energy balls cold. For more extended storage, please keep them in a sealed container in the fridge for up to one week.

Summary:
Nutty Cocoa Energy Balls are a delicious and healthy snack packed with natural ingredients like dates, nuts, and cocoa, providing a perfect energy boost. These balls are easy to prepare and offer a convenient, nutritious snack that is ideal for on-the-go snacking, after workouts, or for a quick energy lift during the day.

Cheesy Kale Chips

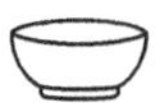  

Ingredients

- 1 large bunch of kale, torn into bite-size pieces (crisp and vibrant)
- 2 tablespoons olive oil (ensures even baking)
- 1/4 cup nutritional yeast (provides a cheesy taste)
- ½ teaspoon garlic powder (for extra zest)
- ½ teaspoon onion powder (deepens the savory notes)
- Salt and freshly ground black pepper (adjust to taste)

Nutritional Information:

Per serving: 150 calories, 6g protein, 13g carbohydrates, 9g fat, 5g fiber, 0mg cholesterol, 300mg sodium, 200mg potassium.

Prep Time: 10 min · Cook Time: 20 min · Serves: 4

Directions

1. **Oven Setup:** Set the oven to 300°F (150°C) and prepare a baking sheet with parchment paper.
2. **Preparing** the kale is a breeze. Mix it with olive oil until each piece is lightly coated. Then, add the nutritional yeast, garlic and onion powders, salt, and pepper, and give it a good toss to ensure a uniform coat.
3. **Baking:** Lay the kale in a single layer on the prepared sheet. Bake for 20 minutes until the edges are crisp but not burnt, flipping halfway through for even cooking.
4. **Cooling:** Remove the kale from the oven and let it sit on the sheet to crisp up further.
5. **Serving:** These are best enjoyed fresh from the oven or stored in an airtight container for a few days to maintain crunch.

Summary:
These **Cheesy Kale Chips** are not just delicious; they're a fantastic snack that combines the health benefits of kale with the indulgent flavor of cheesy seasoning. They are perfect for those seeking a crispy, savory treat without guilt, providing a delicious way to enjoy a nutrient-rich vegetable.

SWEET POTATO CHIPS

Ingredients

- 2 large, sweet potatoes, thinly sliced (sweet and earthy)
- 2 tablespoons olive oil (for a crisp finish)
- Salt and pepper to taste (for seasoning)
- A sprinkle of cinnamon (for a hint of spice)

Nutritional Information:

Per serving: 140 calories, 2g protein, 20g carbohydrates, 7g fat, 3g fiber, 0mg cholesterol, 150mg sodium, 400mg potassium.

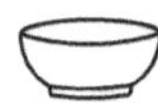  

Prep Time: 10 min   Cook Time: 20 min   Serves: 4

Directions

1. **Prep:** Preheat your oven to 375°F (190°C) and line a baking sheet with parchment paper.
2. **Season:** Coat the sweet potato slices with olive oil, salt, pepper, and a dash of cinnamon, ensuring they are evenly covered.
3. **Arrange:** Lay the slices on the baking sheet in a single layer without overlapping.
4. **Bake:** Bake in the preheated oven for 20 minutes, turning halfway through, until they are crispy and slightly golden.
5. **Serve:** Let the chips cool slightly before serving. Enjoy them as a sweet, crispy treat.

Summary:

Sweet Potato Chips are a delightful snack that offers a healthier alternative to traditional potato chips. These chips are baked, not fried, and seasoned with cinnamon, making them a perfect sweet and savory snack for any occasion. Enjoy sweet potatoes' crisp texture and natural sweetness in a light, crunchy form.

GREEK YOGURT DIP WITH HERBS

Ingredients

- 1 cup Greek yogurt (creamy and tangy)
- 1 tablespoon olive oil (smooth texture)
- 1 tablespoon lemon juice (zesty kick)
- 1 garlic clove, minced (bold flavor)
- 1 tablespoon fresh dill, chopped (refreshing taste)
- 1 tablespoon fresh parsley, chopped (bright and fresh)
- Salt and pepper to taste (seasoning)

Nutritional Information:

Per serving: 100 calories, 6g protein, 6g carbohydrates, 5g fat, 1g fiber, 5mg cholesterol, 150mg sodium, 200mg potassium.

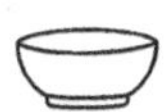  

Prep Time: 10 min   Cook Time: 0 min   Serves: 4

Directions

1. **Mix:** In a bowl, combine the Greek yogurt, olive oil, minced garlic, add lemon juice until smooth and well-blended.
2. **Season:** Add salt and pepper to taste, adjusting the seasoning to your preference.
3. **Garnish:** Stir in the chopped dill and parsley for an added burst of flavor and color.
4. **Serve:** Put the dip to a serving bowl and enjoy with fresh veggies or whole-grain crackers.

Summary:

Greek Yogurt Herb Dip is a refreshing and healthy snack option. The creamy yogurt base, combined with zesty lemon juice and fresh herbs, makes for a delightful dip perfect for any occasion. Enjoy it with crunchy vegetables or whole-grain crackers for a nutritious treat.

Avocado Lime Greek Yogurt Dip

Ingredients

- 1/4 cup chia seeds (for a gelatinous texture and omega-3s)
- 1 ripe avocado, mashed (provides creamy texture)
- 1 cup of plain Greek yogurt (adds tanginess and protein)
- Juice of 1 lime (for zest and freshness)
- 1 clove of garlic, minced (introduces a flavor kick)
- ½ teaspoon salt (for seasoning)
- 1/4 teaspoon black pepper (adds a bit of spice)
- 1 tablespoon of chopped cilantro (optional for herbal freshness)
- A pinch of chili flakes (optional for a spicy edge)

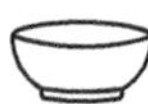

Prep Time: 10 min   Cook Time: 0 min   Serves: 4

Directions

1. **Mix Dip:** In a medium bowl, thoroughly combine mashed avocado, Greek yogurt, lime juice, minced garlic, salt, and black pepper until the mixture is uniformly smooth.
2. **Enhance Flavors:** If using, stir in cilantro and chili flakes to integrate all the flavors.
3. **Chill:** Place the dip in the refrigerator for 30 minutes to blend the flavors, enhancing the tangy and creamy profile.
4. **Serve:** Offer the chilled dip with fresh vegetables like carrots, cucumbers, and bell peppers, or serve with whole-grain crackers.
5. **Garnish:** Optionally, top with additional cilantro or chili flakes before serving for added color and flavor.

Nutritional Information:

Per serving: 120 calories, 6g protein, 8g carbohydrates, 7g fat, 3g fiber, 2mg cholesterol, 310mg sodium, 350mg potassium.

Summary:

This **Avocado Lime Greek Yogurt Dip**, with its creamy avocado, tangy Greek yogurt, and lime zestiness, offers a refreshing flavor that's like a burst of freshness. Whether served with crisp vegetables or whole-grain crackers, this dip is perfect for health-conscious diners looking for a delicious, nutritious snack that will leave them feeling rejuvenated cravings with natural ingredients, making health-conscious individuals feel at ease.

These recipes are designed to be simple yet delicious, ensuring they're accessible to beginners while providing stable energy and helping to maintain healthy blood sugar levels. Enjoy crafting these delightful treats that promise to be as satisfying as they are brilliant for your health.

"Snack Smart" is not just a chapter; it's a guide to a new way of snacking that's both delicious and supportive of your health journey with diabetes. By choosing these snacks, you're treating yourself to tasty bites and nourishing your body with ingredients that won't spike your blood sugar.

Let **"Snack Smart"** be your companion on the path to wellness, one satisfying snack at a time. By making intelligent choices and embracing wholesome ingredients, we've transformed snacking into a joyful experience that nourishes both body and soul. Wave goodbye to guilt and welcome a universe of delicious options with "Snack Smart."

Enjoy snacks that not only please your palate but also enhance your health and happiness.

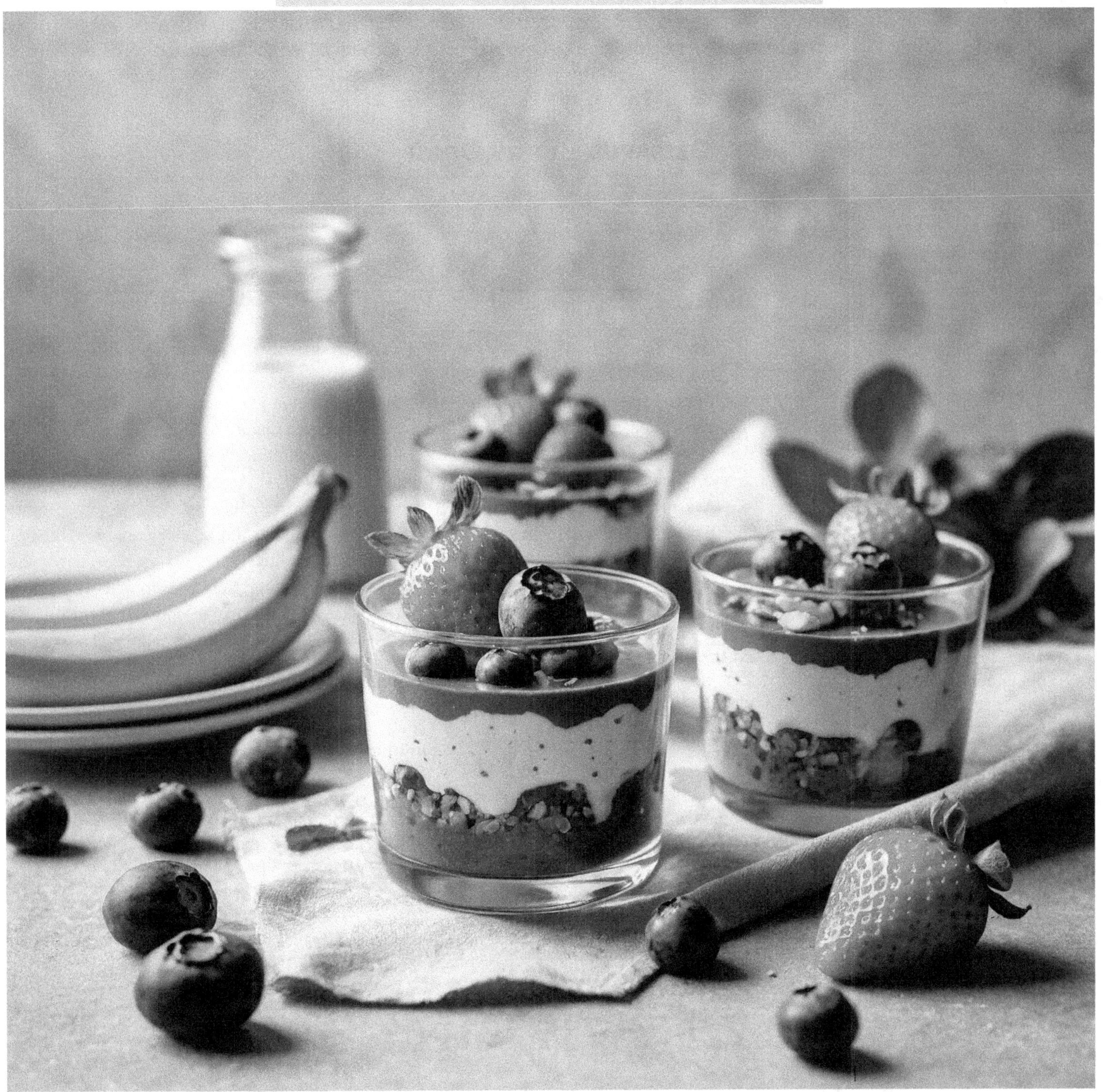

Sweet Endings: Irresistible diabetes-friendly dessert recipes, perfect for special occasions or everyday indulgence.

"Sweet Endings" is not just a cookbook; it's a versatile guide. Including "diabetes-friendly dessert recipes" emphasizes its suitability for individuals with dietary restrictions. Its mention of "special occasions or everyday indulgence" invites readers to explore its versatility. Whether celebrating milestones or satisfying sweet cravings, this cookbook offers a solution for every moment.

85

'**Sweet Endings**' promises an array of delectable treats tailored for individuals managing diabetes, ensuring guilt-free indulgence without compromising flavor. Our recipes are crafted with wholesome ingredients, such as whole grains, natural sweeteners, and fresh fruits, to maintain a balanced nutritional profile. We want to reassure you that you can enjoy desserts without compromising your health. These recipes are not just delicious; they're also good for you.

BLISSFUL BERRY CRISP

Ingredients

- 2 cups of assorted fresh berries, including strawberries, blueberries, and raspberries (packed with vibrant flavors)
- 1 tablespoon of lemon juice (adds a citrusy spark)
- 1/4 cup of granulated erythritol (sweetens without the sugar impact)
- 1/2 cup of old-fashioned rolled oats (provides texture)
- 1/4 cup of almond flour (gives a nutty undertone)
- 2 tablespoons of unsalted butter, melted (brings richness)
- 1/4 teaspoon of ground cinnamon (introduces a warm spice)
- **Optional**: Whipped cream or Greek yogurt (for creaminess), fresh mint leaves (for a fresh accent)

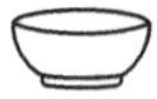  

Prep Time: 15 min   Cook Time: 30 min   Serves: 4

Directions

1. **Oven Setup:** Warm the oven to 350°F (175°C). Lightly grease a baking dish or individual ramekins.
2. **Berry Mixture:** In a bowl, mix the berries with lemon juice and erythritol until evenly coated. Arrange this mixture in your prepared dish or ramekins.
3. **Crumble Creation:** In another bowl, stir the oats, almond flour, butter, and cinnamon until it forms a crumbly mixture.
4. **Assemble:** Evenly distribute the crumble topping over the berries.
5. **Bake:** Place in the oven and cook for roughly 30 minutes until the crumble is golden brown and the fruit mixture has started to bubble.
6. **Serving:** Allow the berry crisp to rest briefly after baking. Serve warm with a scoop of whipped cream or Greek yogurt, and sprinkle fresh mint as an optional garnish.

Nutritional Information:
Per serving: 180 calories, 3g protein, 20g carbohydrates, 10g fat, 5g fiber, 8mg cholesterol, 50mg sodium, 200mg potassium.

Summary:

This **Blissful Berry Crisp** combines succulent berries with a crunchy oat topping, creating a delightful and satisfying dessert that's not overly sweet. The touch of cinnamon and lemon enhances the natural flavors, making it a perfect treat for any occasion. Enjoy it as a cozy dessert that brings the essence of both comfort and freshness to your table.

Velvety Chocolate Avocado Mousse

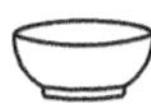  

Ingredients

- 2 ripe avocados (silky and rich)
- 1/4 cup of unsweetened cocoa powder (intensely chocolaty)
- 1/4 cup of powdered erythritol or stevia (cuts the sweetness without sugar)
- 2-3 tablespoons of unsweetened almond milk (adjusts consistency)
- 1 teaspoon of vanilla extract (enhances overall flavor)
- A pinch of salt (sharpens the taste)
- Optional: shaved dark chocolate or fresh berries

Nutritional Information:

Per serving: 150 calories, 4g protein, 10g carbohydrates, 12g fat, 6g fiber, 0mg cholesterol, 50mg sodium, 300mg potassium.

Prep Time: 15 min | Cook Time: 60 min | Serves: 4

Directions

1. **Blend Ingredients:** In a blender, combine the avocados, cocoa powder, erythritol or stevia, almond milk, vanilla extract, and salt. Blend until creamy, scraping down the sides of the blender regularly to incorporate all ingredients.
2. **Adjust Texture:** Gradually mix almond milk into the mousse to thin it to your desired consistency.
3. **Chilling:** Pour the mousse into serving dishes, cover, and chill in the refrigerator for at least an hour to enhance the flavors and texture.
4. **Finish and Serve:** Garnish with shaved chocolate or berries before serving. Enjoy the rich, indulgent taste of this chocolatey delight.

Summary:

Velvety Chocolate Avocado Mousse offers a luscious, guilt-free indulgence that blends the creamy texture of avocado with rich cocoa for a decadent treat. This dessert not only satisfies your chocolate cravings but does so in a healthy and wholesome way. Whether as a dessert or a luxurious snack, this mousse is sure to impress with its creamy texture and deep chocolate flavor.

Lemon Berry Yogurt Parfait

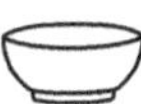  

Ingredients

- 1 cup plain Greek yogurt (creamy and tangy)
- Zest of 1 lemon (for a burst of citrus flavor)
- ``1 tablespoon of fresh lemon juice (for a zesty tang)
- 2 tablespoons powdered erythritol or stevia (for sweetness without the sugar spike)
- 1/2 cup low-carb granola or almond meal (for crunch)
- 1/2 cup fresh mixed berries (such as strawberries, blueberries, raspberries) (juicy and vibrant)
- **Optional toppings**: lemon slices or mint leaves (for garnish)

Prep Time: 10 min | Cook Time: 0 min | Serves: 2

Directions

1. **Prepare Lemon Yogurt:** In a mixing bowl, whisk together the Greek yogurt, lemon zest, lemon juice, and sweetener until smooth. Adjust sweetness as desired.
2. **Layer Parfait:** Alternate layers of lemon yogurt, granola, and mixed berries in two serving glasses or bowls.
3. **Garnish:** Top each parfait with additional berries, lemon slices, or mint leaves for freshness.
4. **Serve:** Enjoy immediately to savor the refreshing blend of tangy yogurt, crunchy granola, and sweet berries.

Nutritional Information:

Per serving: 150 calories, 10g protein, 15g carbohydrates, 6g fat, 3g fiber, 0mg cholesterol, 50mg sodium, 200mg potassium.

Summary:

Delight in the layers of creamy lemon yogurt, crunchy granola, and sweet, juicy berries. This **Lemon Berry Yogurt Parfait** offers a light and refreshing treat, perfect for a quick breakfast, an afternoon snack, or a healthy dessert.

DIVINE DARK CHOCOLATE TRUFFLES

Ingredients

- 6 oz dark chocolate, 70% cocoa, chopped (luxuriously rich)
- 1/2 cup heavy cream (creates smoothness)
- 1 tablespoon unsalted butter (adds silkiness)
- 1/2 teaspoon vanilla extract (flavor enhancer)
- Cocoa powder, unsweetened coconut, or nuts (for coating)

Nutritional Information:
Per serving: 110 calories, 1g protein, 6g carbohydrates, 9g fat, 2g fiber, 5mg sodium

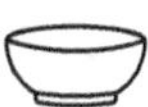  

Prep Time: 15 min   Cook Time: 60 min   Serves: 12 truffles

Directions

1. **Prepare Chocolate Mixture:** Heat cream and butter until simmering. Pour over chocolate, let sit, then stir in vanilla.
2. **Chill:** Refrigerate until firm.
3. **Form Truffles:** Scoop and roll the mixture into balls. Coat in desired toppings.
4. **Chill Again:** Refrigerate truffles to set.
5. **Serve:** Enjoy these divine treats chilled or at room temperature, savoring the deep chocolate flavor.

Summary:

These **Divine Dark Chocolate Truffles** are a true indulgence, offering a rich, melt-in-your-mouth experience. Perfect for any chocolate connoisseur, they provide a satisfying end to any meal or a luxurious treat for special occasions.

VELVETY PUMPKIN SPICE PUDDING

Ingredients

- 1 can (15 oz) pumpkin puree (delivers a deep pumpkin taste)
- 1/2 cup unsweetened almond milk (adds creaminess)
- 1/4 cup powdered erythritol or stevia (ensures sweetness without the calories)
- 2 tablespoons cornstarch (acts as a thickener)
- 1 teaspoon pumpkin pie spice (provides a warm, seasonal flavor)
- 1/2 teaspoon vanilla extract (enhances overall flavor)
- A pinch of salt (sharpens the flavors)
- **Optional:** Sugar-free whipped cream or cinnamon for garnish (adds a decorative touch)

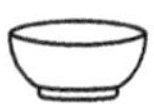  

Prep Time: 10 min   Cook Time: 10 min   Serves: 4

Directions

1. **Prepare Pudding:** Combine all ingredients except the garnish in a medium saucepan. Whisk until smooth.
2. **Cook:** Over medium heat, stir the mixture continuously until it thickens and begins to bubble, about 5-7 minutes.
3. **Simmer:** Turn the heat to low and let simmer for 2-3 minutes to achieve the perfect pudding consistency.
4. **Serve:** Spoon the pudding into bowls or ramekins. Let cool slightly before topping with optional whipped cream or a sprinkle of cinnamon.

Nutritional Information:
Per serving: 80 calories, 1g protein, 15g carbohydrates, 1g fat, 5g fiber, 0mg cholesterol, 50mg sodium, and 300mg potassium.

Summary:

Experience the essence of autumn with this **Creamy Pumpkin Spice Pudding**. This dessert combines rich pumpkin and classic fall spices for a comforting treat. Perfect for a fantastic evening, it offers a delightful finish to any meal without compromising your health goals.

Charming Cherry Almond Tart

Ingredients

For the Crust:

- 1 1/2 cups almond flour (provides a nutty base)
- 1/4 cup coconut flour (enhances texture)
- 1/4 cup powdered erythritol or stevia (adds sweetness)
- 1/4 teaspoon salt (flavor enhancer)
- 1/4 cup unsalted butter, melted (for a rich crust)
- **For the Filling:**
- 2 cups frozen cherries, pitted (full of tartness)
- 2 tablespoons powdered erythritol or stevia (sweetens)
- 1 tablespoon of lemon juice (brightens the flavor)
- 1 tablespoon of almond flour (thickens the filling)
- 1/2 teaspoon almond extract

For the Topping:

1/4 cup sliced almonds, toasted (adds a crunchy texture

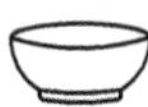  

Prep Time: 20 min | Cook Time: 25 min | Serves: 8

Directions

1. **Preheat Oven:** Set to 350°F (175°C). Prepare a 9-inch tart pan with a removable bottom.
2. **Crust:** Creating the base for our Charming Cherry Almond Tart is a breeze. Simply mix almond and coconut flour with sweetener and salt. Blend in butter to form crumbs. Press into the tart pan. It's that easy!
3. **Filling:** Toss cherries with sweetener, lemon juice, almond flour, and extract. Allow to thaw slightly.
4. **Assemble Tart:** Pour cherry mixture into the crust. Top with almonds.
5. **Bake:** 25-30 minutes until bubbling and golden. Cool on a wire rack.
6. **Serve:** Garnish with whipped cream or mint, if desired. This sumptuous tart features a rich blend of tart cherries and crunchy almonds.

Nutritional Information: **Per serving:** 200 calories, 4g protein, 15g carbohydrates, 15g fat, 4g fiber, 50mg sodium.

Summary:
Take a bite of the **Charming Cherry Almond Tart,** where the tartness of the cherries dances with the sweetness of the crunchy topping, creating a symphony of tastes and textures that's sure to leave you wanting more.

Divine Angel Food Cake

Ingredients

- 1 cup all-purpose flour (light and airy)
- 1 1/2 cups powdered erythritol or stevia (for sweetness without the sugar spike)
- 12 large egg whites, room temperature (for fluffy texture)
- 1 1/2 teaspoons cream of tartar (for stability)
- 1 teaspoon of vanilla extract
- 1/4 teaspoon salt
- Optional toppings: fresh berries or sugar-free whipped cream (for garnish)

Nutritional Information:
Per serving: 100 calories, 5g protein, 20g carbohydrates, 0g fat, 0g fiber, 0mg cholesterol, 150mg sodium, 100mg potassium.

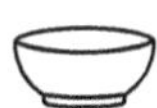  

Prep Time: 20 min | Cook Time: 40-45 min | Serves: 8

Directions

1. **Preheat Oven:** Set it to 350°F (175°C) and position the rack in the middle.
2. **Prepare Pan:** Sift flour and half the sweetener into an ungreased tube pan; set aside.
3. **Whip Egg Whites:** Beat egg whites with cream of tartar, vanilla, and salt to soft peaks. Gradually add the remaining sweetener, beating to stiff, glossy peaks.
4. **Fold in Flour:** Carefully fold the flour mixture into egg whites in three parts to keep the volume.
5. **Transfer Batter:** Smooth the batter into the prepared pan and level the top.
6. **Bake:** Cook until the cake is golden and springs back when touched.
7. **Invert to Cool:** Invert the pan onto a cooling rack; cool completely.
8. **Unmold:** Loosen the cake with a knife and transfer it to a plate.
9. **Serve:** Cut into slices and serve with optional fresh berries or whipped cream.

Summary:
Enjoy the heavenly texture and light sweetness of this **Divine Angel Food Cake**. It's the perfect dessert for any gathering, offering all the joy of a delicious treat without the guilt. Pair it with fresh berries or a dollop of whipped cream for an elegant serving.

WHOLESOME NUTTY BANANA BREAD

Ingredients

- 1 1/2 cups almond flour (for a nutty flavor)
- 1/2 cup coconut flour (adds moisture)
- 1 teaspoon of baking soda (helps the bread rise)
- 1/4 teaspoon salt (enhances the flavors)
- 3 ripe bananas, mashed (adds natural sweetness)
- 3 large eggs (bind the ingredients)
- 1/4 cup unsweetened almond milk (adds moisture)
- 1/4 cup coconut oil, melted (provides richness)
- 1/4 cup powdered erythritol or stevia (sweetens without sugar)
- 1 teaspoon of vanilla extract (for flavor depth)
- 1/2 cup chopped walnuts or pecans (adds texture)
- Optional: 1/4 cup sugar-free chocolate chips, one teaspoon ground cinnamon

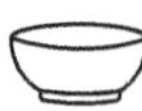

Prep Time: 15 min   Cook Time: 50-60 min   Serves: 1 loaf

Directions

1. **Prepare:** Preheat the oven to 350°F (175°C) and grease a 9x5-inch loaf pan.
2. **Mix Dry Ingredients:** In a large bowl, whisk together almond flour, coconut flour, baking soda, and salt.
3. **Combine Wet Ingredients:** In another bowl, blend mashed bananas, eggs, almond milk, melted coconut oil, sweetener, and vanilla.
4. **Mix Wet and Dry:** Stir wet ingredients into dry, fold in nuts and any optional add-ins.
5. **Bake:** Pour batter into the prepared pan and bake for 50-60 minutes.
6. **Cool:** Let bread cool in the pan before transferring to a rack.
7. **Enjoy** Slice and serve, possibly with coffee or as dessert.

Nutritional Information:
Per serving: 200 calories, 6g protein, 15g carbohydrates, 14g fat, 4g fiber, 150mg sodium.

Summary:

This **Wholesome, Nutty Banana Bread** offers a delightful, healthy twist on traditional banana bread. It incorporates the rich flavors and textures of nuts and bananas. Perfect for a comforting snack or breakfast, this moist, flavorful bread is perfect any time of the day.

Ingredients

Shortcake:

- 1 1/2 cups almond flour (nutty flavor)
- 1/4 cup coconut flour (adds moisture)
- 1/4 cup powdered erythritol or stevia (sweetens without sugar)
- 1 teaspoon of baking powder (leavening agent)
- 1/4 teaspoon salt (flavor enhancer)
- 1/4 cup unsweetened almond milk (adds moisture)
- 1/4 cup coconut oil, melted (richness)
- 2 large eggs (bind ingredients)
- 1 teaspoon of vanilla extract (enhances flavor)

Strawberry Topping:

- 2 cups fresh strawberries, sliced (vibrant and juicy)
- 1 tablespoon of powdered erythritol or stevia (adds sweetness)
- 1 teaspoon of lemon juice (adds brightness)

Whipped Topping:

- 1 cup heavy cream, chilled (creamy texture)
- 1 tablespoon of powdered erythritol or stevia (sweetens)
- 1/2 teaspoon vanilla extract
- Optional: Fresh mint, sugar-free chocolate shavings

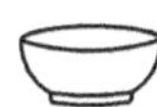  

Prep Time: 15 min   Cook Time: 15min   Serves: 6

Directions

1. **Preheat Oven:** Set oven to 350°F (175°C). Prepare a baking sheet.
2. **Make Shortcake:** Mix dry ingredients; combine wet ingredients in another bowl. Mix to form a dough.
3. **Shape and Bake:** Form dough into rounds on a baking sheet and bake until golden.
4. **Prepare Topping:** Mix strawberries with sweetener and lemon juice.
5. **Whip Cream:** Whip cream with sweetener and vanilla to stiff peaks.
6. **Assemble:** Layer shortcakes with strawberries and whipped cream.
7. **Garnish and Serve:** Add mint or chocolate if desired and serve.

Nutritional Information:
Per serving: 250 calories, 5g protein, 20g carbohydrates, 18g fat, 6g fiber, 100mg sodium.

Summary:

Enjoy the **Sensational Strawberry Shortcake**, a fresh and delightful take on a classic dessert. This treat, layered with light almond flour cakes, lush strawberries, and a cloud of whipped cream, melds complex flavors into a perfect finale for any meal. Ideal for summer gatherings or as a special treat, this shortcake promises a satisfyingly sweet experience without the sugar spike.

DREAMY COCONUT MANGO SORBET

Ingredients

- 2 ripe mangoes peeled and diced (packed with tropical sweetness)
- 1 can (14 oz) coconut milk (ensures a creamy texture)
- 1/4 cup powdered erythritol or stevia (for a guilt-free sweetness)
- 1 tablespoon lime juice (adds a zesty note)
- A sprinkle of salt (enhances the sweet flavors)
- Optional: Unsweetened shredded coconut for garnish (adds texture)

Nutritional Information:

Per serving: 150 calories, 1g protein, 20g carbohydrates, 8g fat, 3g fiber, 0mg cholesterol, 50mg sodium, and 300mg potassium.

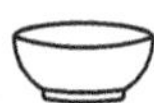  

Prep Time: 10 min   Freeze Time: 4 hours   Serves: 4

Directions

1. **Blend Ingredients:** In a blender, combine mangoes, coconut milk, sweetener, lime juice, and salt. Blend until smooth.
2. **Adjust Flavor:** Taste and tweak the sweetness or tartness, if necessary.
3. **Freeze:** Transfer to an ice cream maker or a shallow dish. If using a dish, freeze and stir occasionally to prevent ice crystals.
4. **Serve:** Once firm, scoop and serve in bowls, topped with shredded coconut if desired.

Summary:

Dive into a refreshingly sweet escape with this **Coconut mango sorbet**. The vibrant blend of mango and coconut offers an indulgent and refreshing tropical taste, perfect for a warm day or as a light dessert. This sorbet is delicious and a health-conscious choice that can be enjoyed without any dietary guilt.

COCOA-DUSTED ALMOND TRUFFLES

Ingredients

- 1 cup almonds (rich and crunchy)
- 1/2 cup dates (natural sweetener)
- 2 tbsp cocoa powder (for dusting)

Nutritional Information:

Per serving: 150 calories, 4g protein, 15g carbohydrates, 9g fat, 3g fiber.

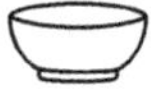  

Prep Time: 20 min   Chill Time: 60 min   Serves: 6

Directions

1. **Blend** and process almonds and dates until the mixture forms a sticky dough.
2. **Shape:** Roll into small balls and coat with cocoa powder.
3. **Chill:** Refrigerate until firm.

Summary:

Cocoa-dusted almond Truffles are a decadent treat. Rich almonds and sweet dates are dusted in cocoa, combining to create a perfect bite-sized delight for any chocolate lover.

LUSCIOUS LEMON-BERRY PARFAIT

Ingredients

- 1 cup creamy Greek yogurt, tangy delight
- Zest of a sun-kissed lemon for a citrus burst
- 1 spoon of lemon juice, zingy and fresh
- 2 tablespoons of a sugar-free sweetener, like erythritol or stevia, for guiltless sweetness
- 1/2 cup of crunchy granola or nutty almond meal
- 1/2 cup of a juicy berry medley, strawberries, blueberries, raspberries
- Garnish options: thin lemon slices or fresh mint leaves for a decorative flair

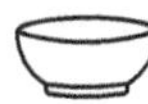  

Prep Time: 10 min   Cook Time: 0 min   Serves: 2

Directions

1. **Whip** the Greek yogurt with lemon zest and juice and sweeten with your choice of sugar alternative to creamy perfection.
2. In charming glasses, **artistically layer** the zesty yogurt, granola, or almond meal and a cascade of berries.
3. **Garnish** with a lemon wheel or a mint leaf atop for a picturesque finish.
4. **Dive** into this enchanting parfait, a symphony of zesty, tangy, and sweet notes.

Nutritional Information:
Per serving: 150 calories, 10g protein, 0g carbohydrates, 6g fat.

Summary:
Indulge in the vibrant dance of tart lemon and sweet berries nestled between layers of hearty granola crunch. This **Lemon-Berry Parfait** isn't just a treat; it's a journey through a garden of delights, a refreshing escapade that's both nourishing and exhilarating. The zing of the lemon, the burst of the berries, and the crunch of the granola create a symphony of flavors that will leave you craving for more. Get ready for a taste explosion.

SWEET PEACH CRUMBLE

Ingredients

- 4 cups of fresh, juicy peaches, sliced
- 1 teaspoon of cinnamon (for a hint of spice)
- 1/2 a cup of rolled oats (for texture)
- 1/4 cup of almond flour (adds a nutty flavor)
- 2 tablespoons of coconut oil melted (for moisture)
- 1/4 cup of erythritol or stevia (for sweetness)

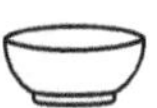  

Prep Time: 15 min   Cook Time: 30 min   Serves: 4

Directions

1. **Heat It**: Preheat the oven to 350°F (175°C) and grease a baking dish.
2. **Arrange Peaches**: Place the peach slices evenly in the dish and dust with cinnamon.
3. **Crumble Together**: Combine oats, almond flour, coconut oil, and erythritol until crumbly.
4. **Bake to Perfection**: Distribute the crumble mixture uniformly over the peaches and bake until the surface turns golden and the mixture starts bubbling around 30 minutes.
5. **Cool and Serve**: Allow the crumble to cool slightly before serving, letting the flavors meld.

Nutritional Information:
Per serving: 180 calories, 3g protein, 23g carbohydrates, 9g fat, 4g fiber, 0mg cholesterol, 10mg sodium, 300mg potassium.

Summary:
Experience the simplicity of the **Sweet Peach Crumble**, where each bite perfectly blends spiced, juicy peaches and a crispy oat topping. This dessert brings a comforting warmth, making it ideal for a sweet end to any meal or a cozy afternoon treat.

Raspberry Almond Delight Bars

Ingredients

- 2 cups fresh raspberries (tart and vibrant)
- 1 cup almond flour (for a rich, nutty base)
- 1/3 cup unsweetened shredded coconut (adds texture)
- 1/4 cup sliced almonds (for a crunchy finish)
- 3 tablespoons coconut oil (binds the mix)
- 2 tablespoons of erythritol or stevia (for natural sweetness).

Nutritional Information:

Per serving: 180 calories, 4g protein, 20g carbohydrates, 10g fat, 5g fiber, 0mg cholesterol, 10mg sodium, 200mg potassium.

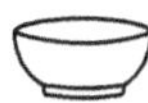  

Prep Time: 10 min   Cook Time: 25 min   Serves: 6

Directions

1. **Preheat and Prep**: Set the oven to 350°F (175°C) and prepare an 8-inch square baking pan with parchment paper.
2. **Layer Base**: Combine almond flour, coconut, and one tablespoon of sweetener; press into the pan's base.
3. **Assemble**: Spread raspberries over the base and sprinkle with another tablespoon of sweetener.
4. **Add Crunch**: Top with sliced almonds and bake until the almonds are toasted and raspberries are bubbling, about 25 minutes.
5. **Cool and Enjoy**: Let the bars cool before slicing and serving.

Summary:

Indulge in the guilt-free **Raspberry Almond Delight Bars,** a fusion of sweet and tart flavors balanced with a crunchy almond topping. This easy-to-make treat is perfect for those seeking a light yet satisfying dessert or a healthy snack.

Chocolate Almond Ricotta Mousse

Ingredients

- 1 cup ricotta cheese (for creaminess)
- 1/4 cup unsweetened cocoa powder (rich chocolate flavor)
- 1/4 cup powdered erythritol or stevia (adds sweetness without the sugar spike)
- 1/4 cup chopped almonds (adds texture and nuttiness)
- 1 teaspoon vanilla extract (enhances flavor)

Nutritional Information:

Per serving: 20 calories, 12g protein, 10g carbohydrates, 15g fat, 3g fiber, 35mg cholesterol, 80mg sodium, 200mg potassium.

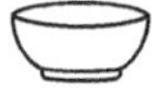  

Prep Time: 10 min   Cook Time: 1 hour   Serves: 4

Directions:

1. **Blend the Mixture:** In a mixing bowl, blend together ricotta cheese, cocoa powder, sweetener, and vanilla extract. Using an electric mixer, whip until the mixture is smooth and has a velvety texture.
2. **Add Crunch:** Fold the chopped almonds into the chocolate mixture to introduce a delightful crunch.
3. **Chill:** Transfer the mousse to serving dishes and refrigerate for at least one hour to allow the flavors to meld and the texture to firm up.
4. **Serve:** Enjoy this rich and creamy mousse as a luxurious dessert that healthily satisfies your chocolate cravings.

Summary:

Indulge in the sumptuous flavors of **Chocolate Almond Ricotta Mousse,** a creamy and satisfying treat that combines the richness of chocolate with the lightness of ricotta and the crunch of almonds. This dessert is perfect for a decadent finish to any meal, offering a guilt-free way to enjoy a diabetic-friendly sweet treat.

TROPICAL COCONUT RICE PUDDING

Ingredients

- 1 cup of Arborio rice (for a creamy texture)1 can of coconut milk (rich and tropical; use a vegan alternative if desired)1/4 cup shredded coconut (for added flavor and texture)
- 1/4 cup erythritol or stevia (for a guilt-free sweetness)
- 1 teaspoon vanilla extract (flavor enhancer)
- Fresh mango and pineapple diced (for a fresh, fruity topping).

Nutritional Information:

Per serving: 200 calories, 3g protein, 30g carbohydrates, 7g fat, 2g fiber, 0mg cholesterol, 50mg sodium, 200mg potassium.

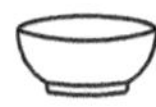  

Prep Time: 10 min   Cook Time: 25 min   Serves: 4 servings (4 cup)

Directions

1. **Cook Rice**: Combine rice, coconut milk, and half the sweetener in a saucepan. Cook until the rice is soft and creamy, about 25 minutes.
2. **Enhance Flavor**: Stir in vanilla extract and the remaining sweetener, adjusting to taste.
3. **Prepare Toppings**: While the rice cooks dice the mango and pineapple.
4. **Serve with a Tropical Twist**: Spoon the warm rice pudding into bowls, top with fresh mango, pineapple, and a sprinkle of shredded coconut.

Summary:

Tropical Coconut Rice Pudding is a creamy delight that whisks your taste buds away to a sun-kissed beach. Each spoonful is a harmonious blend of lush coconut and aromatic vanilla, crowned with vibrant tropical fruits. Indulge in this dessert as a sweet finale to any meal or as a decadent treat.

CHOCOLATE PEANUT BUTTER BANANA BITES

Ingredients

- 2 large bananas (sweet and creamy)
- 1/4 cup natural peanut butter (smooth and rich)
- 1/2 cup dark chocolate chips, melted (intense chocolate flavor)
- 1/4 teaspoon sea salt (flavor enhancer)

Nutritional Information:

Per serving: 180 calories, 4g protein, 20g carbohydrates, 10g fat, 3g fiber, 0mg cholesterol, 100mg sodium, 250mg potassium.

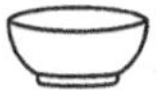  

Prep Time: 15 min   Cook Time: 60 min   Serves: 6

Directions

1. **Prepare Bananas**: Slice bananas into rounds about 1/2 inch thick.
2. **Add Filling**: Spoon a small peanut butter onto half the banana slices. Top with the remaining slices, making little sandwiches.
3. **Dip in Chocolate**: Dip half of each banana sandwich into melted chocolate, then set them on a parchment-lined baking sheet.
4. **Freeze for Perfection**: Sprinkle with sea salt and freeze until firm, about 1 hour.

Summary:

Chocolate Peanut Butter Banana Bites are the epitome of indulgence, making a delightful snack or dessert. These frozen treats offer a satisfying crunch from frozen bananas, the richness of peanut butter, and the decadent pleasure of dark chocolate—a guaranteed hit for all ages.

BERRY DELIGHT SMOOTHIE BOWL

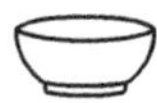

Ingredients

- 1 cup frozen mixed berries (bright and tangy)
- 1/2 banana (natural sweetness)
- 1/2 cup Greek yogurt (creamy texture)
- Toppings: fresh berries, nuts (added crunch and nutrients)

Nutritional Information:
Per serving: 120 calories, 6g protein, 18g carbohydrates, 3g fat, 4g fiber.

Prep Time: 5 min | Cook Time: 0 min | Serves: 2

Directions

1. **Blend**: Process berries, banana, and yogurt until smooth.
2. **Garnish**: Pour into bowls and top with fresh berries and nuts.

Summary:

Berry Delight Smoothie Bowl is bursting with fresh flavors and vibrant colors, making it a perfect energizing start to your day or a refreshing snack.

ALMOND AND BERRY CHIA PUDDING

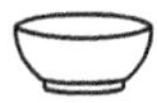

Ingredients

- 1/4 cup chia seeds
- 1 cup unsweetened almond milk
- 1 teaspoon vanilla extract
- 2 tablespoons powdered erythritol or stevia
- 1/2 cup mixed berries (fresh or thawed from frozen)
- 2 tablespoons slivered almonds

Nutritional Information:

Per serving: 150 calories, 4g protein, 15g carbohydrates, 9g fat, 7g fiber, 0mg cholesterol, 50mg sodium, 200mg potassium.

Prep Time: 10 min (plus chilling) | Cook Time: 0 min | Serves: 4

Directions

1. **Combine** chia seeds, almond milk, vanilla, and sweetener in a bowl.
2. **Stir** thoroughly to combine, then let sit for 5 minutes.
3. **Blend** well to eliminate clumps, then cover and chill in the refrigerator for at least 2 hours, or overnight, until it sets into a pudding.
4. **Top** with berries and slivered almonds before serving.

Summary:

Almond and Berry Chia Pudding offer a delightful combination of nutty almonds and sweet, succulent berries enveloped in luscious chia seed pudding. Not only does this dish excite the taste buds, but it also delivers substantial nutritional benefits. Packed with fiber, protein, and healthy fats, it's a guilt-free treat perfect for any moment you crave a luxurious yet wholesome indulgence.

SPICED PEAR AND YOGURT PARFAIT

Ingredients

- 2 large pears, diced (sweet and slightly tangy)
- 1 teaspoon ground cinnamon (warm spice)
- 1 cup Greek yogurt (thick and creamy)
- 1/4 cup granola (crunchy texture)
- 1 tablespoon honey (natural sweetness)

Nutritional Information:

Per serving: 150 calories, 6g protein, 22g carbohydrates, 4g fat, 3g fiber, 5mg cholesterol, 50mg sodium, 200mg potassium.

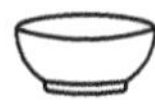  

Prep Time: 10 min   Cook Time: 25 min   Serves: 4 servings (4 cup)

Directions

1. **Cook Pears**: In a skillet, sauté pears with cinnamon until tender and aromatic, about 5 minutes.
2. **Layer Parfait**: In serving glasses, layer Greek yogurt, cooked pears, and granola.
3. **Drizzle and Serve**: Drizzle honey over each parfait before serving.

Summary:

Spiced Pear and Yogurt Parfaits marries the comforting warmth of spiced pears with the cool, creamy embrace of Greek yogurt, all topped with a satisfying crunch of granola. It's a flavorful and nutritious dessert or breakfast option that layers textures and tastes for a truly delightful eating experience.

SILKY PUMPKIN PIE CUSTARD

Ingredients

- 1 can pumpkin puree (smooth and flavorful)
- 2 eggs (binds the custard)
- 1/4 cup erythritol or stevia (sweet without sugar)
- 1 tsp pumpkin pie spice (seasonal spices)
- 1 tsp vanilla extract (flavor depth)

Nutritional Information:

Per serving: 90 calories, 3g protein, 10g carbohydrates, 4g fat, 2g fiber.

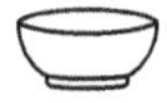  

Prep Time: 10 min   Cook Time: 30 min   Serves: 4

Directions

1. **Mix Ingredients**: Whisk together pumpkin puree, eggs, sweetener, pumpkin pie spice, and vanilla.
2. **Bake**: Pour into ramekins and bake at 350°F until set, about 30 minutes.
3. **Chill and Serve**: Let excellent, then refrigerate before serving.

Summary:

Silky Pumpkin Pie Custard offers a taste of autumn with each spoonful, providing a light, creamy dessert that's comforting and satisfying without the crust.

MINT CHOCOLATE CHIP FROZEN YOGURT

Ingredients

- 2 cups Greek yogurt (creamy and tangy)
- 1/4 cup of chopped fresh mint leaves (adds a refreshing flavor)
- 1/2 cup dark chocolate chips (rich and decadent)

Nutritional Information:

Per serving: 80 calories, 6g protein, 20g carbohydrates, 8g fat, 2g fiber.

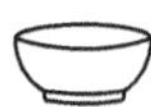 Prep Time: 10 min

 Freeze Time: 2 hours

 Serves: 4 servings

Directions

1. **Blend:** Mix Greek yogurt with chopped mint and chocolate chips until well combined.
2. **Freeze:** Pour the mixture into a container and freeze until firm.
3. **Serve:** Scoop and serve immediately for a refreshing treat.

Summary:

Mint Chocolate Chip Frozen Yogurt offers a delightful twist on traditional ice cream. It blends tangy yogurt with fresh mint and decadent chocolate chips for a refreshing and satisfying dessert.

CARAMELIZED FIG AND RICOTTA TOAST

Ingredients

- 4 slices of whole-grain bread (hearty and fiber-rich)
- 1 cup ricotta cheese (smooth and creamy)
- 8 figs, halved and caramelized (sweetly indulgent)
- A drizzle of honey (natural sweetness)
- 1/4 cup chopped pistachios (for a crunchy finish)

Nutritional Information:

Per serving: • 250 calories, 10g protein, 35g carbohydrates, 10g fat, 5g fiber.

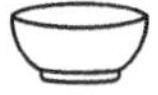 Prep Time: 5 min

 Cook Time: 10 min

 Serves: 4

Directions

1. **Prepare:** Toast the bread slices to a golden crisp.
2. **Assemble:** Spread ricotta on each slice, top with caramelized figs, and drizzle with honey.
3. **Garnish:** Sprinkle chopped pistachios over the top.
4. **Serve:** Enjoy this luxurious toast warm.

Summary:

Caramelized Fig and Ricotta Toast combines the lushness of sweet figs with creamy ricotta on a crunchy toast base, drizzled with honey and sprinkled with pistachios, creating a decadent yet easy-to-make dessert.

Espresso Hazelnut Biscotti

Ingredients

- 1 cup almond flour (for a low-carb structure)
- 1/4 cup granulated sugar substitute, like stevia, monk fruit, or other (sweetness without the sugar spike)
- 1/2 cup roasted hazelnuts, chopped (adds texture and nutty flavor)
- 1 tablespoon espresso powder (for a rich coffee flavor)
- 2 large eggs (helps bind the ingredients)
- 1/2 teaspoon vanilla extract (enhances flavor)
- 1/4 teaspoon salt (balances sweetness)

Nutritional Information:

Per serving: 150 calories, 6g protein, 8g carbohydrates, 12g fat, 3g fiber

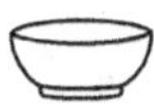  

Prep Time: 20 min   Bake Time: 40 min   Serves: 8 servings

Directions

1. **Mix Ingredients:** In a large bowl, combine almond flour, erythritol, chopped hazelnuts, espresso powder, salt, eggs, and vanilla extract. Stir until the mixture forms a cohesive dough.
2. **Shape the Dough:** On a parchment-lined baking sheet, shape the dough into a log about 12 inches long and 2 inches wide.
3. **First Bake:** Place in a preheated oven at 350°F (175°C) and bake for 25 minutes or until the log is firm to the touch.
4. **Cool and Slice:** Remove from the oven and let cool for 10 minutes. Using a serrated knife, cut the log diagonally into 1/2-inch thick slices.
5. **Second Bake:** Arrange the slices back on the baking sheet and return to the oven for 15 minutes, turning halfway through to ensure even crispness.
6. **Cool and Serve:** Let the biscotti cool completely on a rack before serving. They will continue to crisp as they cool.

Summary:

Enjoy a delightful **Espresso Hazelnut Biscotti**, perfectly tailored for those managing diabetes. These biscotti offer a sophisticated crunch with a hint of espresso, making them an excellent choice for a low-carb, sugar-free treat alongside your favorite coffee or tea.

Pineapple Ginger Sorbet

Ingredients

- 3 cups fresh pineapple, chopped (tropical and sweet)
- 1 tbsp fresh ginger, grated (spicy and pungent)
- Juice of 1 lime (adds zestiness)

Nutritional Information:

Per serving: • 00 calories, 1g protein, 25g carbohydrates, 0g fat, 2g fiber

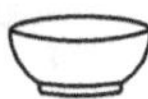  

Prep Time: 10 min   Freeze Time: 3 hours   Serves: 4

Directions

1. **Blend:** Puree the pineapple, ginger, and lime juice until smooth.
2. **Freeze:** Place the blended mix into an ice cream machine, lay it flat in a dish, and freeze until it sets.
3. **Serve:** Scoop the sorbet into bowls and serve immediately.

Summary:

Pineapple Ginger Sorbet is a refreshingly icy treat that melds the sweet juiciness of pineapple with the zing of fresh ginger, topped off with a dash of lime. This simple yet exotic sorbet is perfect for cooling down on a hot day or as a light dessert after a meal.

"**Sweet Endings**" offers a range of delicious and easy dessert recipes. These recipes are ideal for individuals managing diabetes or those seeking healthier dessert options. From smooth and creamy mousse to crunchy truffles, each recipe is designed to be a breeze, ensuring a satisfying finish to any meal. **Enjoy these recipes, knowing they bring a wholesome conclusion to your culinary explorations with minimal effort.**

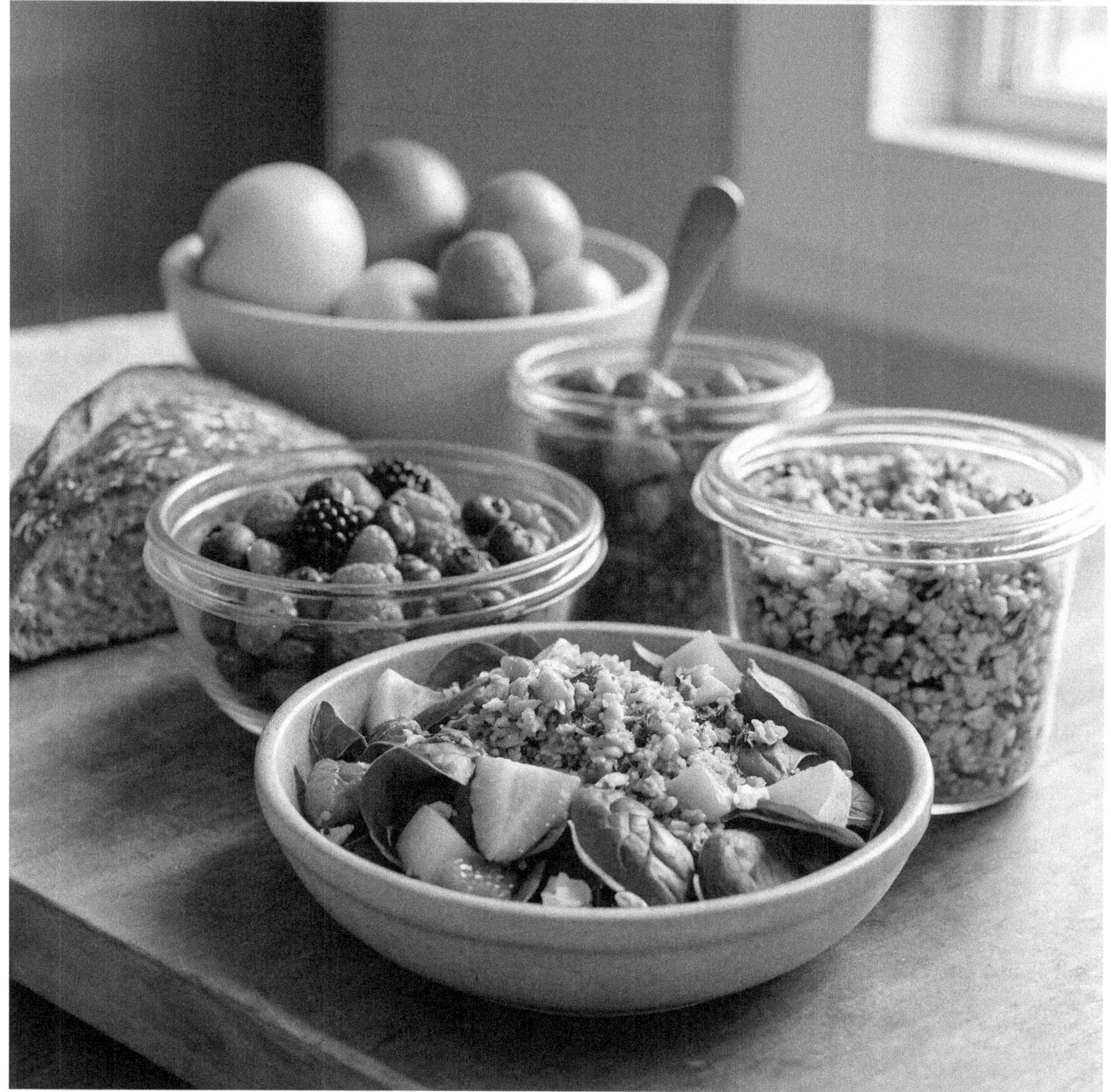

Welcome to your 30-Day Meal Plan from the Delicious Diabetic Cookbook for Beginners.

This comprehensive guide is designed to help you manage prediabetes and Type 2 diabetes with ease and enjoyment. Over the next month, you'll embark on a culinary journey, introducing you to various flavors and ingredients while keeping your health in check.

Here's a 30-day meal plan tailored from the recipes provided in your file. It is designed to offer a variety of delicious, diabetes-friendly breakfast, lunch, dinner, and dessert meals. The meal plan is divided into four weeks, starting with a foundation-building week and followed by three weeks aimed at establishing healthy eating habits.

The plan starts with **"Kickstart Your Journey,"** a week to establish a strong foundation in diabetic-friendly eating habits. Here, you'll explore simple yet flavorful dishes that will set the tone for the coming weeks.

As you progress to **"Building Healthy Habits"** from weeks 2 to 4, you'll diversify your palate with an exciting mix of recipes that ensure every meal is healthy but also delicious and satisfying. From hearty breakfasts to sumptuous dinners and delightful desserts, each recipe is tailored to fit a diabetic diet without sacrificing taste.

This meal plan is more than just a schedule; it's a stepping stone toward a healthier lifestyle. It includes meal preparation and grocery shopping tips to streamline your cooking process and effortlessly fit healthy eating into your daily routine.

Let's get started on this path to improved health and delicious dining!

WEEK 1: KICKSTART YOUR JOURNEY.

This week-long meeting builds a solid foundation for healthy eating habits.

Day	Breakfast	Lunch	Dinner	Dessert
1	Mediterranean Shakshuka	Avocado Chicken Salad	Garlic Lemon Chicken Stir-Fry	Blissful Berry Crisp
2	Peanut Butter Banana Bowl	Quinoa Veggie Wrap	Herb-Crusted Salmon	Velvety Chocolate Avocado Mousse
3	Antioxidant Acai Bowl	Turmeric Lentil Soup	Baked Cod with Olives and Tomatoes	Lemon Berry Yogurt Parfait
4	Hearty Oatmeal Creations	Caprese Zoodle Salad	Vegetable Lasagna	Divine Dark Chocolate Truffles
5	Cinnamon Apple Oatmeal	Tuna and White Bean Salad	Thai Beef Salad	Velvety Pumpkin Spice Pudding
6	Green Goddess Bowl	Turkey and Apple Sandwich	Mushroom and Spinach Risotto	Charming Cherry Almond Tart
7	Chocolate Hazelnut Oatmeal	Roasted Veggie Hummus Wrap	Turkey Chili	Divine Angel Food Cake

Three weeks of structured meal plans featuring a variety of recipes from the book, with tips for meal prep and grocery shopping.

Day	Breakfast	Lunch	Dinner	Dessert
8	Veggie Omelette	Chickpea Greek Salad	Cauliflower Steak	Wholesome Nutty Banana Bread
9	Egg Muffins with Feta and Spinach	Soba Noodle Salad with Peanut Dressing	Grilled Shrimp Tacos	Sensational Strawberry Shortcake
10	Berry Yogurt Parfait	Butternut Squash Soup	Zucchini Noodle Pad Thai	Dreamy Coconut Mango Sorbet
11	Tropical Yogurt Parfait	Mediterranean Chickpea Salad	Pumpkin Curry	Cocoa-Dusted Almond Truffles
12	Apple Pie Parfait	Spinach and Feta Stuffed Chicken Breast	Eggplant Parmesan	Luscious Lemon-Berry Parfait
13	Peanut Butter Chocolate Parfait	Cold Asian Noodle Salad	Chicken Cacciatore	Sweet Peach Crumble
14	Chia Seed Pudding Parfait	Lentil and Sweet Potato Chili	Beef Stir-Fry with Broccoli	Raspberry Almond Delight Bars
15	Quinoa Breakfast Bowl	Cauliflower Rice Stir-Fry	Portobello Mushroom Burgers	Chocolate Almond Ricotta Mousse
16	Sweet Potato Hash	Stuffed Bell Peppers	Spaghetti Squash and Meatballs	Tropical Coconut Rice Pudding
17	Avocado Chickpea Toast	Kale and White Bean Soup	Asian Chicken Lettuce Wraps	Chocolate Peanut Butter Banana Bites
18	Zucchini Pancakes	Vegan Taco Salad	Pesto Pasta with Sun-Dried Tomatoes	Berry Delight Smoothie Bowl
19	Breakfast Salad	Ratatouille with Grilled Chicken	Tofu and Vegetable Stir-Fry	Almond and Berry Chia Pudding
20	Grilled Vegetable Quinoa Bowl	Creamy Pumpkin Soup	Roast Beef and Vegetables	Spiced Pear and Yogurt Parfait
21	Vegetarian Lettuce Wraps Recipe	Shrimp and Avocado Salad	Grilled Chicken Caesar Salad	Silky Pumpkin Pie Custard
22	Almond Butter Banana Wraps	Balsamic Beet and Goat Cheese Salad	Butternut Squash Risotto	Blissful Berry Crisp
23	Veggie Breakfast Burritos	Smoked Salmon and Avocado on Rye	Vegetarian Chili	Velvety Chocolate Avocado Mousse
24	Apple Sandwiches	Mango Chicken Salad	Pork Tenderloin with Apples	Lemon Berry Yogurt Parfait
25	Breakfast Smoothie	Curried Tofu Salad	Garlic Butter Baked Salmon	Divine Dark Chocolate Truffles
26	Oatmeal Breakfast Bars	Avocado Lime Greek Yogurt Dip	Roasted Turkey Breast with Herb Vegetables	Velvety Pumpkin Spice Pudding

Day	Breakfast	Lunch	Dinner	Dessert
27	Weekend Brunch Specials	Spiced Chickpea Crunchies	Spicy Tofu and Vegetable Curry	Charming Cherry Almond Tart
28	Sweet Potato Waffles	Cucumber Rolls with Hummus	Nutty Cocoa Energy Balls	Divine Angel Food Cake
29	Zesty Lemon Yogurt Parfait	Mediterranean Shakshuka	Savory Oatmeal with Avocado	Espresso Hazelnut Biscotti
30	Chia Seed Pudding with Mixed Berries	Grilled Chicken Salad with Avocado and Walnut	Baked Salmon with Steamed Broccoli and Quinoa	Mint Chocolate Chip Frozen Yogurt

As we conclude the 30-day meal plan adventure in the **"Delicious Diabetic Cookbook for Beginners,"** we hope it has sparked a love for healthy, balanced eating and given you the tools to manage prediabetes and type 2 diabetes effectively.

This journey was designed to introduce you to many delicious, diabetes-friendly recipes that satisfy your taste buds, nourish your body, and stabilize your blood sugar levels.

From the foundational first week of kickstarting healthy habits to the last three weeks of building and solidifying those habits, each recipe was chosen to inspire and facilitate a sustainable lifestyle change.

Keep exploring these recipes and integrating them into your daily life as you continue your path to wellness and vitality.

Remember, each meal is a step towards a healthier, more flavorful you!

HANDY HELPERS: SIMPLIFYING YOUR CULINARY JOURNEY

Dive into your culinary journey with confidence and the right tools at your fingertips, simplifying meal planning and grocery shopping. This section explores valuable tips and tricks to make healthy cooking a breeze and a comprehensive pantry staples list to keep your kitchen stocked with nutritious essentials. Prepare to enhance your cooking skills and discover the pleasures of crafting tasty, diabetes-friendly dishes.

- **Pantry Staples List**: Ensure your kitchen is always ready for culinary creativity with these essential pantry staples:
- **Whole grains:** Stock up on brown rice, quinoa, oats, and whole wheat pasta.
- **Legumes:** Stock up on various canned or dried beans and lentils to enrich your soups, salads, and stews with high-protein goodness.
- **Healthy fats:** Choose healthy fats like olive oil, avocado oil, and coconut oil for cooking and dressings, and enjoy nuts and seeds as snacks or garnishes.
- **Herbs and Spices:** Enhance your meals by adding a vibrant array of dried herbs and spices such as basil, oregano, turmeric, and cinnamon to elevate their flavors.
- **Low-sodium Broth:** Use vegetable or chicken broth to deepen the flavors of your soups, sauces, and stir-fries without adding too much sodium.
- **Canned tomatoes:** Use diced or crushed tomatoes as a base for sauces, stews, and chili recipes.
- **Nut butter:** Enjoy the versatility of almond butter, peanut butter, or sunflower seed butter for spreads, dips, and smoothies.
- **Vinegar:** For salad dressings and marinades, keep apple cider, balsamic, and white vinegar on hand.
- **Sweeteners:** Embrace natural sweeteners such as honey, maple syrup, or stevia to sweeten your dishes judiciously.
- **Non-dairy milk:** Choose unsweetened almond, soy, or coconut milk for dairy-free alternatives in recipes and beverages.
- **Meal Prep Tips:** Make meal preparation a breeze with these simple tips and strategies:
- **Planning:** Dedicate weekly time to planning meals and compiling a shopping list from your recipes, eliminating last-minute hassles.
- **Batch cooking:** Prepare large batches of staple ingredients such as grains, proteins, and roasted vegetables for multiple weekly meals.
- **Portion control:** Use portion-sized containers to divide meals into individual servings for easy grab-and-go options and portion control.
- **Label and date:** Label and date meal containers to ensure freshness and avoid food waste.
- **Freeze for later:** Freeze leftover soups, stews, and casseroles in meal-sized portions for convenient heat-and-eat meals on busy days.

With the right tools and resources, meal planning and preparation can become a seamless and enjoyable part of your healthy lifestyle. By stocking your pantry with nutritious staples and implementing time-saving meal prep techniques, you'll be well-equipped to create delicious and diabetes-friendly meals easily.

Say goodbye to kitchen stress and hello to culinary confidence as you embrace **Handy Helpers' convenience** in your cooking journey.

CHAPTER 11: CONCLUSION

As you reach the end of this cookbook, take a moment to celebrate every step you've taken towards a healthier, happier you. Each recipe you've tried, every nutritious meal you've savored, is a testament to your commitment to better health.

But remember, this is just the beginning of your journey. Keep that determination burning bright as you continue making small, sustainable lifestyle changes. Whether swapping out unhealthy ingredients for nutritious alternatives or finding new ways to enjoy your favorite foods guilt-free, every choice brings you closer to your wellness goals.

Let this cookbook be your guide, source of inspiration, and constant companion on this journey of self-discovery and empowerment. With each delicious dish you prepare, you're not just nourishing your body; you're nourishing your spirit, too.

So, keep going strong, pushing forward, and never forget the incredible power you hold to shape your health destiny. Your journey of encouragement has only just begun, and the possibilities are endless. Here's to a future filled with health, happiness, and endless culinary adventures. Cheers to you and the delicious life that awaits, where you are the master of your health journey.

Remember, you are the captain of your health ship, steering it towards a healthier, happier you.

CELEBRATE YOUR SUCCESS

Celebrate Your Journey to Health

In the pages of this cookbook, you've embarked on a flavorful voyage toward better health and well-being. As you close the book, take a moment to reflect on the journey you've undertaken. Celebrate every recipe you've mastered, every nutritious ingredient you've embraced, and every step you've taken toward a healthier lifestyle.

Your dedication and commitment to adopting healthier habits deserve recognition. You've shown resilience, determination, and willingness to prioritize your health; you should be proud. Each meal you've prepared nourishes your body and spirit, fueling you with the energy and vitality needed to thrive.

So, take a moment to pat yourself on the back, revel in your achievements, and recognize your significant progress.

As you progress, remember that success lies in reaching your goals and the journey. Embrace the challenges, savor the victories, and cherish every moment. Your trip to health is not just about the destination; it's about the transformative power of self-discovery and growth. Each step you take, each meal you prepare, is a testament to your commitment to better health. So, celebrate your journey, for it's as beautiful as it is delicious, and it's a journey that's uniquely yours. And remember, this is just the beginning of your story. There are countless more recipes to explore, adventures to embark on, and victories to celebrate.

So, keep cooking, exploring, and embracing the delicious journey ahead, knowing your potential for growth and discovery is limitless.

KEEP GOING STRONG ON YOUR DELICIOUS JOURNEY

As you close the pages of this cookbook, remember that your path to better health is more like a marathon than a sprint. It's about making small, sustainable changes that gradually improve your well-being. While you've already taken significant steps towards healthier eating habits, the path ahead is filled with opportunities for growth, discovery, and continued progress.

It's essential to keep the momentum going, stay committed to balanced nutrition principles, and make choices that support your health and vitality. Each meal is an opportunity to nourish yourself; every ingredient is a step towards health.

But staying on track means something other than sacrificing flavor or enjoyment. It's quite the opposite. By embracing this cookbook's delicious recipes and wholesome ingredients, you've discovered that eating well can be satisfying and enjoyable. So, continue to savor the flavors, experiment with new dishes, and delight in the culinary experiences that await you.

Challenges are a part of the journey, not a reason to give up. It's not about being perfect but about making steady progress. Treat yourself kindly, cherish your achievements, and see each challenge as a chance to improve and strengthen your resolve towards better health. Every setback is a step forward in disguise.

As you navigate the ups and downs of your journey, know that you're not alone. Draw strength from your community, seek support from loved ones, and remember that you have the power to overcome any obstacle that comes your way.

So, Keep going! Your courage and resilience can conquer any challenge. Your journey towards better health is a testament to your strength and commitment to living your best life. As you continue this delicious path, may you find joy, fulfillment, and lasting wellness every step of the way.

EMBRACE YOUR JOURNEY OF ENCOURAGEMENT

As you reflect on the pages of this cookbook, remember that your journey toward better health is not just about the food you eat—it's about the choices you make and the mindset you cultivate. It's a journey of empowerment, of harnessing the power within you to make positive changes and transform your life for the better.

Each recipe you've explored, each meal you've savored, is a step forward on your path to wellness. But beyond the ingredients and cooking techniques lies a more profound journey of self-discovery, self-care, and self-empowerment.

This cookbook taught you that taking control of your health isn't about restriction or deprivation. It's about abundance—nutritious foods, flavor, and possibilities for a vibrant, fulfilling life.

So, as you continue your journey, remember to be kind to yourself. Celebrate your successes, no matter how small. Acknowledge your challenges and use them as opportunities for growth. Above all, believe in yourself and your ability to create the life you deserve. Let each day be a new opportunity to nourish your body, nurture your spirit, and live your best life.

So, dear reader, embrace this journey with courage, grace, and a heart full of hope. For in the journey of encouragement lies the power to transform your life and create the future you've always dreamed of.

DIABETIC-FRIENDLY TIPS FOR EATING OUT AND ENJOYING SOCIAL EVENTS:

- **Preview the Menu**

Before heading out, take a moment to preview the menu online. This simple step can help you identify dishes rich in vegetables, lean proteins, and whole grains, allowing you to make more informed and healthier choices.

- **Smart Swaps**

To control your intake, choose steamed, grilled, or baked dishes instead of fried ones. Request dressings and sauces on the side.

- **Portion Probing**

Consider sharing a meal or setting aside half to take home. This strategy helps manage portion sizes but also assists in controlling carb counts, which is crucial for maintaining your blood sugar levels.

- **Hydration Hints**

Choose water or unsweetened beverages over sugary drinks. If you drink alcohol, do so in moderation and with food.

- **Mindful Munching**

Practice mindful eating by savoring each bite and eating slowly. This approach allows your body to signal fullness, promoting better digestion and preventing overeating.

- **Dessert Decisions**

Share dessert with the table or choose fresh fruit if you desire dessert.

- **Speak Up**

Feel free to ask how dishes are prepared and request modifications to fit your dietary needs.

- **Plan Ahead**

If you know you'll be dining out, adjust your meals earlier in the day to accommodate.

- **Stay Balanced**

Try to keep your meals balanced with carbs, proteins, and fats.

- **Enjoy the Experience**

Embrace the joy of dining out and the vibrant social aspect it brings. Remember, enjoying the company is just as important as the meal. With these practical tips, you can enjoy dining out and celebrating life's special moments while staying true to your health goals. Dive into each social occasion confidently, knowing you can navigate any menu.

INDEX

A

B

C

D

E